Guidelines on

Optimal feeding of low birth-weight infants in low-and middle-income countries

2011

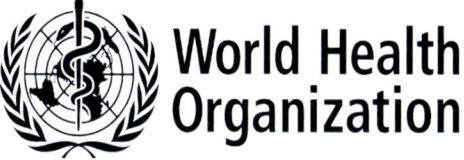

WHO Library Cataloguing-in-Publication Data

Guidelines on optimal feeding of low birth-weight infants in low- and middle-income countries.

1.Infant nutrition. 2.Infant, Low birth weight. 3.Nutritional requirements. 4.Feeding methods. 5.Infant food. 6.Guidelines. 7.Developing countries. I.World Health Organization.

ISBN 978 92 4 154836 6   (NLM classification: WS 120)

© World Health Organization 2011

CONTENTS

Annexes

1   **Detailed GRADE profiles summarizing evidence**

2   **Summary of individual research studies which formed the basis of recommendations**

ACKNOWLEDGEMENTS

Many individuals made significant contributions to the development of these guidelines. Ramesh Agarwal, Zulfiqar Bhutta, Karen Edmond, Sandra Lang, Indira Narayanan, Samuel Newton, Vinod Paul, Muhammad Sohail Salat, María Asunción Silvestre, Nalini Singhal and Anthony Williams served as members of the Guidelines Development Group. WHO staff members involved included: Rajiv Bahl, Carmen Casanovas, Bernadette Daelmans, Ornella Lincetto, Jeevasankar Mari, Jose Martines and Randa Saadeh. Felicity Savage King participated in writing the draft guidelines; Peggy Henderson edited the final draft.

I

ABBREVIATIONS AND GLOSSARY

CI	Confidence interval
CLD	Chronic lung disease
DARE	Cochrane database of abstracts of reviews of effectiveness
dl	Decilitre
ELBW	Extremely low birth weight
ES	Effect size
g	Gram
GDG	Guideline development group
GRADE	System for grading the quality of evidence and the strength of recommendations
HIV	Human immunodeficiency virus
IMCI	Integrated management of childhood illness
IMPAC	Integrated management of pregnancy and childbirth
IQ	Intelligence quotient
i.u.	International unit
kg	Kilogram
l	Litre
LBW	Low birth weight
mg	Milligram
ml	Millilitre
MD	Mean difference
NEC	Necrotizing enterocolitis
OR	Odds ratio
Palladai	Cup with a beak
PICO	Population, intervention, comparison, outcome
RCT	Randomized controlled trial
RDA	Recommended daily allowance
ROP	Retinopathy of prematurity
RR	Relative risk
SD	Standard deviation
SGA	Small for gestational age
TPN	Total parenteral nutrition
VLBW	Very low birth weight
WHO	World Health Organization
WMD	Weighted mean difference

EXECUTIVE SUMMARY

Low birth weight (LBW) has been defined by the World Health Organization (WHO) as weight at birth less than 2500 g. The global prevalence of LBW is 15.5%, which means that about 20.6 million such infants are born each year, 96.5% of them in developing countries. There is significant variation in LBW rates across the United Nations regions, with the highest incidence in South-Central Asia (27.1%) and the lowest in Europe (6.4%).

LBW can be a consequence of preterm birth (defined as birth before 37 completed weeks of gestation), or due to small size for gestational age (SGA, defined as weight for gestation <10th percentile), or both. In addition, depending on the birth weight reference used, a variable but small proportion of LBW infants are born at term and are not SGA. Intrauterine growth restriction, defined as a slower than normal rate of fetal growth, is usually responsible for SGA. LBW thus defines a heterogeneous group of infants: some are born early, some are born at term but are SGA, and some are both born early and SGA.

Being born with LBW is generally recognized as a disadvantage for the infant. LBW infants are at higher risk of early growth retardation, infectious disease, developmental delay and death during infancy and childhood.

Countries can substantially reduce their infant mortality rates by improving the care of LBW infants. Experience from developed and low- and middle-income countries has clearly shown that appropriate care of LBW infants, including feeding, temperature maintenance, hygienic cord and skin care, and early detection and treatment of complications, can substantially reduce mortality in this highly vulnerable group. Interventions to improve feeding are likely to improve the immediate and longer-term health and well-being of the individual infant and have a significant impact on neonatal and infant mortality levels in the population. Better feeding was one of the first interventions for preterm babies in the 1960s in the United Kingdom and was associated with reduced case fatality in hospitals before the advent of intensive care.

The objective of these guidelines is to improve the quality of care received by LBW infants in developing countries through improved capacity of health workers. These guidelines focus on the feeding of clinically stable LBW infants in low-and middle income countries. They do not specifically address the feeding of infants with a birth weight less than 1.0 kg (known as extremely LBW, ELBW), who are often clinically unstable and may require parenteral nutrition. Guidance on the management of clinically unstable infants is addressed in other WHO documents.

The guideline development group identified 18 research questions to be of the highest priority for development of recommendations. Most of the questions are relevant to all LBW infants (birth weight less than 2.5 kg) but some are specific to very LBW (VLBW) infants (birth weight less than 1.5 kg). The questions do not specifically address ELBW infants. For each question, the following four outcomes were considered to be critical: *mortality, severe morbidity, neurodevelopment and anthropometric status*. Benefits and harms in critical outcomes formed the basis of the recommendations for each question.

Studies from developing and developed countries that included infants with a birth weight less than 2500 g or gestation less than 37 weeks were considered for inclusion in this review. Efforts were made to identify relevant non-English language articles and abstracts also.

A standardized form was used to extract relevant information from studies. Systematically extracted data included: study identifiers, setting, design, participants, sample size, intervention or exposure, control or comparison group, outcome measures and results. The following quality characteristics were recorded for all studies: allocation concealment or risk of selection bias (observational studies), blinding of intervention or observers or risk of measurement bias, loss to follow up, intention to treat analysis or adjustment for confounding factors, and analysis adjusted for cluster randomization (the latter only for cluster-randomized controlled trials, RCTs).

We used a modified GRADE approach for assessing the quality of evidence and the recommendations (for details, see **Methodology** section). The quality of the set of included studies reporting results for an outcome was graded as: high, moderate, low or very low.

The strength of a recommendation reflects the degree of confidence that the desirable effects of adherence to a recommendation outweigh the undesirable effects. The decisions were made on the basis of evidence of benefits and harms; quality of evidence; values and preferences of policy-makers, health-care providers and parents; and whether costs are qualitatively justifiable relative to benefits in low- and middle- income countries.

Each recommendation was graded as *strong* when there was confidence that the benefits clearly outweigh the harms, or *weak* when the benefits probably outweigh the harms, but there was uncertainty about the trade-offs. A strong or weak recommendation was further classified as *situational* if the benefits outweigh the harms in some situations but not in others. For example, some recommendations were considered relevant only to settings in low- and middle-income countries where resources were very limited (e.g. Recommendations 3, 4, 5 and 12) while others were considered relevant only to settings where certain types of facilities were available (e.g. Recommendations 2 and 17).

2011 WHO Recommendations on optimal feeding of low-birth-weight infants

No.	Recommendation*	Type of recommendation	Quality of evidence (at least 1 critical outcome)
	What to feed?		
	a. Choice of milk		
1.	Low-birth-weight (LBW) infants, including those with very low birth weight (VLBW), should be fed mother's own milk.	*Strong*	*Moderate*
2.	LBW infants, including those with VLBW, who cannot be fed mother's own milk should be fed donor human milk (recommendation relevant for settings where safe and affordable milk-banking facilities are available or can be set up).	*Strong situational*	*High*
3.	LBW infants, including those with VLBW, who cannot be fed mother's own milk or donor human milk should be fed standard infant formula (recommendation relevant for resource-limited settings). VLBW infants who cannot be fed mother's own milk or donor human milk should be given preterm infant formula if they fail to gain weight despite adequate feeding with standard infant formula.	*Weak situational*	*Low*
4.	LBW infants, including those withVLBW, who cannot be fed mother's own milk or donor human milk should be fed standard infant formula from the time of discharge until 6 months of age (recommendation relevant for resource-limited settings).	*Weak situational*	*Low*
5.**	VLBW infants who are fed mother's own milk or donor human milk should not routinely be given bovine milk-based human-milk fortifier (recommendation relevant for resource-limited settings). VLBW infants who fail to gain weight despite adequate breast-milk feeding should be given human-milk fortifiers, preferably those that are human milk based.	*Weak situational*	*Low*
	b. Supplements		
6.**	VLBW infants should be given vitamin D supplements at a dose ranging from400 i.u to 1000 i.u. per day until 6 months of age.	*Weak*	*Very low*
7.**	VLBW infants who are fed mother's own milk or donor human milk should be given daily calcium (120-140 mg/kg per day) and phosphorus (60-90 mg/kg per day) supplementation during the first months of life.	*Weak*	*Low*
8.**	VLBW infants fed mother's own milk or donor human milk should be given 2-4 mg/kg per day iron supplementation starting at 2 weeks until 6 months of age.	*Weak*	*Low*
9.	Daily oral vitamin A supplementation for LBW infants who are fed mother's own milk or donor human milk is not recommended at the present time, because there is not enough evidence of	*Weak*	*Low*

	benefits to support such a recommendation.		
10.	Routine zinc supplementation for LBW infants who are fed mother's own milk or donor human milk is not recommended at the present time, because there is not enough evidence of benefits to support such a recommendation.	*Weak*	*Moderate*
When and how to initiate feeding?			
11.	LBW infants who are able to breastfeed should be put to the breast as soon as possible after birth when they are clinically stable.	*Strong*	*Low*
12.**	VLBW infants should be given 10 ml/kg per day of enteral feeds, preferably expressed breast milk, starting from the first day of life, with the remaining fluid requirement met by intravenous fluids (recommendation relevant for resource-limited settings).	*Weak situational*	*Low*
Optimal duration of exclusive breastfeeding			
13.	LBW infants should be exclusively breastfed until 6 months of age.	*Strong*	*Low*
How to feed?			
14.	LBW infants who need to be fed by an alternative oral feeding method should be fed by cup (or *palladai,* which is a cup with a beak) or spoon.	*Strong*	*Moderate*
15.**	VLBW infants requiring intragastric tube feeding should be given bolus intermittent feeds.	*Weak*	*Low*
16.**	In VLBW infants who need to be given intragastric tube feeding, the intragastric tube may be placed either by oral or nasal route, depending upon the preferences of health-care providers.	*Weak*	*Very low*
How frequently to feed and how to increase the daily feed volumes?			
17.	LBW infants who are fully or mostly fed by an alternative oral feeding method should be fed based on infants' hunger cues, except when the infant remains asleep beyond 3 hours since the last feed (recommendation relevant to settings with an adequate number of health-care providers).	*Weak situational*	*Moderate*
18**	In VLBW infants who need to be fed by an alternative oral feeding method or given intragastric tube feeds, feed volumes can be increased by up to 30 ml/kg per day with careful monitoring for feed intolerance.	*Weak*	*Moderate*

* None of the recommendations address sick LBW infants and infants with birth weight less than 1.0 kg.

** These recommendations specifically address infants with birth weight between 1.0 and 1.5 kg.

INTRODUCTION

Low birth weight (LBW) has been defined by the World Health Organization (WHO) as weight at birth of less than 2.5 kg. The global prevalence of LBW is 15.5%, which amounts to about 20 million LBW infants born each year, 96.5% of them in developing countries.[I]

LBW can be a consequence of preterm birth (before 37 completed weeks of gestation), small size for gestational age (SGA, defined as weight for gestation less than 10th percentile), or a combination of both. Intrauterine growth retardation, defined as slower than normal velocity of fetal growth, is usually responsible for SGA. The term "LBW" thus includes a heterogeneous group of infants: some who are born early, some who are born at term but SGA, and some who are both born early and SGA.

Being born with LBW is generally recognized as a disadvantage for the infant. Preterm birth is a direct cause of 27% of the 4 million neonatal deaths that occur globally every year.[II] Preterm birth and SGA are also important indirect causes of neonatal deaths. Directly or indirectly, LBW may contribute to 60% to 80% of all neonatal deaths.[II] LBW infants are at higher risk of early growth retardation, infection, developmental delay and death during infancy and childhood.[III-IV]

Countries can reduce their neonatal and infant mortality rates by improving the care of LBW infants. Experience from developed and low- and middle-income countries has clearly shown that appropriate care of LBW infants, including their feeding, temperature maintenance, hygienic cord and skin care, and early detection and treatment of problems such as infections can substantially reduce mortality. Interventions to improve feeding are likely to improve the immediate and longer-term health and well-being of the individual infant and have a significant impact on neonatal and infant mortality at a population level. In the 1960s in the United Kingdom, better feeding was one of the first interventions for preterm babies that was associated with reduced case fatality in hospital settings before the advent of intensive care.[V] Kangaroo Mother Care for LBW infants weighing less than 2 kg, which includes exclusive and frequent breastfeeding in addition to skin-to-skin contact and support for the mother-infant dyad, has been shown to reduce mortality in hospital-based studies in low- and middle-income countries.[VI] Studies from India have shown that improved care of LBW infants in the community can be highly effective in improving their survival.[VII-VIII]

LBW infants can be classified according to their gestation into **term** (born after 37 and before 42 completed weeks of gestation) and **preterm** (born up to 37 completed weeks of gestation). Infants in each of these categories can be further divided into two groups based on whether or not they are **SGA**. LBW infants are classified as very low birth weight (VLBW) if their birth weight is less than 1.5 kg, and as extremely low birth weight (ELBW) if their birth weight is less than 1 kg. Preterm infants of less than 32 weeks gestation are at greatest mortality risk, followed by preterm infants of 32-36 weeks gestation who are also SGA, preterm infants of 32-36 weeks gestation who are not SGA, and term LBW infants. All these groups have a higher mortality risk than infants who do not have LBW.

WHO guidelines for feeding of LBW infants have not been available. The quality of care received by LBW infants in many low- and middle-income countries is inadequate. These infants are often not breastfed and many times not fed at all in the first hours and days of life. The objective of these guidelines is to improve the quality of care received by LBW infants through improved capacity of the health workers who care for these infants.

These guidelines were developed using funding to the Department of Maternal, Newborn, Child and Adolescent Health from the United States Agency for International Development. The guidelines will be reviewed and updated in 2014, i.e. three years from the date of their publication.

Guideline Development Group

The following external experts were involved in the development of these guidelines: **African Region**: Juliet Mwanga and Samuel Newton; **Region of the Americas**: Indira Narayanan and Nalini Singhal; **South-East Asia Region**: Ramesh Agarwal and Vinod Paul; **European Region**: Karen Edmond, Sandra Lang and Anthony Williams; **Eastern Mediterranean Region**: Muhammad Sohail Salat and Zulfiqar Bhutta; **Western Pacific Region**: María Asunción Silvestre. None of the members of this Guideline Development Group (GDG) declared any conflicts of interest.

The WHO working group consisted of the following staff members: **Child and Adolescent Health**[1]: Rajiv Bahl, Bernadette Daelmans, Jeevasankar Mari and Jose Martines; **Making Pregnancy Safer**: Ornella Lincetto; **Nutrition for Health and Development**: Carmen Casanovas and Randa Saadeh.

The GDG met once to review the evidence synthesized in a technical review[2]. The WHO working group and a consultant (Felicity Savage King) developed the draft guidelines based on this evidence. This draft was reviewed electronically by the GDG members and approved by them. In 2008-9 these guidelines were field-tested in health facilities in Ghana, India, Pakistan and Uganda. The evidence synthesis was updated by the WHO secretariat (Jeevasankar Mari, Rajiv Bahl and Jose Martines) in the second half of 2010, and the GRADE process was used for classifying the quality of evidence and for development of recommendations. The updated evidence synthesis and several drafts of the revised guidelines were circulated and electronically reviewed by the GDG and finalized by consensus.

---

[1] The Departments of Child and Adolescent Health and Development and Making Pregnancy Safer were merged in 2010 as the Department for Maternal, Newborn, Child and Adolescent Health.
[2] WHO. *Optimal feeding of low-birth-weight infants: technical review.* Geneva, WHO, 2006.

SCOPE OF THE GUIDELINES

Target audience

The primary audience for these guidelines is intended to be health-care workers in first-level health facilities and referral hospitals. However, the guidelines are expected to be used by policy-makers, programme managers and health-facility managers to set up a system for optimal care of LBW infants. Further, many of the recommendations will be relevant for community health workers providing care to LBW infants at home. The information in these guidelines will be included in several capacity strengthening courses for health workers, such as for Essential Newborn Care and Integrated Management of Childhood Illness (IMCI), and in community health worker training on caring for the newborn at home.

Population of interest

The guidelines focus on the feeding of clinically stable LBW infants in low- and middle-income countries. Some of the questions and recommendations focus only on VBLW infants (birth weight less than 1.5 kg). They do not specifically address the feeding of infants with a birth weight less than 1.0 kg (ELBW), who are often clinically unstable and may require parenteral nutrition. Guidance on the management of clinically unstable infants is addressed in other WHO documents.[IX, X] Further, the guidelines do not provide separate recommendations for the two groups of LBW infants, preterm and SGA, because of lack of evidence.

Critical outcomes

Four outcomes were considered to be critical by the guideline development group: ***mortality, severe morbidity, neurodevelopment*** and ***anthropometric status***. Mortality and severe morbidity over the short term (e.g. during initial hospital stay after birth) or longer term (e.g. infant mortality) were considered to be critical. However, neurodevelopment and anthropometric status were considered critical only if measured at age 6 months or more. Benefits and harms in critical outcomes formed the basis of the recommendations. When information on critical outcomes was not available, other non-critical outcomes were considered. Examples of these other outcomes include breastfeeding duration or exclusivity, short-term growth, duration of hospital stay, haemoglobin levels and bone mineralization.

Priority questions

These guidelines address the following questions that were identified to be of the highest priority, expressed in PICO (Population, Intervention, Comparison, Outcome) format:

What should LBW infants be fed?

1. In LBW infants (P), what is the effect of feeding mother's own milk (I) compared with feeding infant formula (C) on critical outcomes - *mortality, severe morbidity, neurodevelopment and anthropometric status* (O)?

2. In LBW infants who cannot be fed mother's own milk (P), what is the effect of feeding donor human milk (I) compared with feeding infant formula (C) on critical outcomes (O)?

3. In LBW infants who cannot be fed mother's own milk or donor human milk (P), what is the effect of feeding preterm infant formula (I) compared with feeding standard infant formula (C) on critical outcomes (O)?

4. In LBW infants who cannot be fed mother's own milk or donor human milk (P), what is the effect of feeding nutrient-enriched infant formula from hospital discharge until 6 months of age (I) compared with feeding standard infant formula (C) on critical outcomes (O)?

5. In VLBW infants who are fed mother's own milk or donor human milk (P), what is the effect of multi-component fortification of breast milk (I) compared with no fortification of breast milk (C) on critical outcomes (O)?

6. In VLBW infants who are fed mother's own milk or donor human milk (P), what is the effect of giving 2-4 Recommended Daily Allowance (RDA) of vitamin D supplements (I) compared with 1 RDA of vitamin D supplements (C) on critical outcomes (O)?

7. In VLBW infants who are fed mother's own milk or donor human milk (P), what is the effect of calcium and phosphorus supplementation (I) compared with no supplementation (C) on critical outcomes (O)?

8. In VLBW infants who are fed mother's own milk or donor human milk (P), what is the effect of starting iron supplementation at 2 weeks of age (I) compared with starting iron supplementation at 2 months of age (C) on critical outcomes (O)?

9. In VLBW infants who are fed mother's own milk or donor human milk (P), what is the effect of daily oral vitamin A supplementation (I) compared with no supplementation (C) on critical outcomes (O)?

10. In LBW infants who are fed mother's own milk or donor human milk (P), what is the effect of zinc supplementation (I) compared with no supplementation (C) on critical outcomes (O)?

When should feeding be initiated in LBW infants?

11. In LBW infants who are able to breastfeed (P), what is the effect of initiation of breastfeeding in the first day of life (I) compared with delaying breastfeeding for more than 24 hours (C) on critical outcomes (O)?

12. In VLBW infants born in settings where total parenteral nutrition is not possible (P), what is the effect of starting small amounts of oral feeds (about 10 ml/kg per day) in the first few days of life (I) compared with no enteral feeding (C) on critical outcomes (O)?

What should be the duration of exclusive breastfeeding for LBW infants?

13. In LBW infants (P), what is the effect of exclusive breastfeeding for 6 months (I) compared with an exclusive breastfeeding duration of 4 months or less (C) on critical outcomes (O)?

How should LBW infants be fed?

14. In LBW infants who need to be fed by an alternative oral feeding method (P), what is the effect of feeding by a cup or *palladai* [cup with a beak] (I) compared with bottle-feeding (C) on critical outcomes (O)?

15. In VLBW infants who need to be given intragastric tube feeding (P), what is the effect of bolus intermittent feeding (I) compared with continuous feeding (C) on critical outcomes (O)?

16. In VLBW infants who need to be given intragastric feeding (P), what is the effect of orogastric tube feeding (I) compared with nasogastric tube feeding (C) on critical outcomes (O)?

How much and how frequently should LBW infants be fed?

17. In LBW infants who are fully or mostly fed by an alternative oral feeding method (P), what is the effect of feeding based on infants' hunger cues (I) compared with strict scheduled feeding (C) on critical outcomes (O)?

18. In VLBW infants who need to be fed by an alternative oral feeding method or given intragastric feeds (P), what is the effect of rapid ($\geq$30 ml/kg per day) progression of feeds (I) compared with slow ($\leq$20 ml/kg per day) progression (C) on critical outcomes (O)?

METHODOLOGY

Evidence synthesis

Search strategy

A series of systematic reviews were conducted and published by WHO as *Optimal feeding of low-birth-weight infants: technical review* in 2006. The databases searched included the Cochrane database of systematic reviews of RCTs, the Cochrane controlled trials register, the Cochrane database of abstracts of reviews of effectiveness (DARE), the Cochrane neonatal collaborative review group specialized register, MEDLINE (1966 to 2005), and EMBASE (1966 to 2005). The reference lists of relevant articles and a number of key journals were hand searched. Every effort was made to include relevant non-English language articles and abstracts. This approach was complemented by an additional search in August-September 2010 to identify relevant research papers published between January 2005 and August 2010. The first set of search terms ("all fields" and "MESH terms") was related to the population of interest: LBW infant, preterm infant, premature infant, SGA infant, fetal growth retardation, intrauterine growth retardation, intrauterine growth restriction. The studies identified also needed to have at least one of the search terms in the second set related to issues in feeding of LBW infants. The second set of search terms included: feeding, enteral nutrition, breastfeeding, breast milk, human milk, donor milk, formula, human-milk fortifier, vitamin, micronutrient, vitamin A, vitamin D, calcium, phosphorus, zinc, iron, cup, bottle, spoon, tube, feeding tolerance, trophic feeding, minimal enteral nutrition and gut priming.

Data abstraction and summary tables of individual studies

A standardized form was used to extract information from relevant studies. Systematically extracted data included: study identifiers, setting, design, participants, sample size, intervention or exposure, control or comparison group, outcome measures and results. The following quality characteristics were recorded for RCTs: allocation concealment, blinding of intervention or observers, loss to follow-up, intention to treat analysis, analysis adjusted for cluster randomization (the latter only for cluster-RCTs). The quality characteristics recorded for observational studies were likelihood of reverse causality, selection bias and measurement bias, loss to follow-up and analysis adjusted for confounding.

The studies were stratified according to the type of intervention or exposure, study design, birth weight and gestational age, where possible. Effects were expressed as relative risks (RR) or odds ratios (OR) for categorical data, and as mean differences (MD) or weighted mean differences (WMD) for continuous data where possible. Where results adjusted for potential confounders were available, particularly for observational studies, they were used in preference to unadjusted results. Where results adjusted for potential confounders were not available, unadjusted results were used. All studies reporting on a critical outcome were summarized in a table of individual studies (see **Annexes**).

Pooled effects

Pooled effects for developing recommendations were considered, wherever feasible. If results of three or more RCTs were available for an outcome, and the overall quality of evidence using the GRADE approach was at least "low", observational studies were not considered. However, if there were less than three RCTs for an outcome or the quality of evidence was "very low", the effects from RCTs were pooled with those from available cohort and case-control studies.

Pooled effects from published systematic reviews were used if the meta-analysis was appropriately done, and the reviews were up to date. However, if any relevant published study not included in the systematic review or a methodological problem with the meta-analysis was identified, the results were pooled using the "metan" command in Stata 11.0. For pooling, the author-reported adjusted effect sizes and confidence intervals (CIs) were used as far as possible. Random effects models for meta-analysis were used if there was important inconsistency in effects, and the random effects model was not unduly affected by small studies. Where pooling of results was not possible, the range of effect sizes observed in the individual studies was used in the development of recommendations.

Grading the quality of evidence

A modified GRADE approach for assessing the quality of evidence was used. The quality of the set of included studies reporting results for an outcome was graded as: high, moderate, low or very low. The interpretation of the grades in these guidelines is:

High: One can be sure that the intervention is beneficial, has no effect or is harmful. The results, including the magnitude of the pooled effect, are unlikely to change with new studies.

Moderate: One can be reasonably sure that the intervention is beneficial, has no effect or is harmful. However, the magnitude of the pooled effect may change with new studies.

Low: Although it is likely that the intervention is beneficial, has no effect or is harmful, one cannot be sure. The magnitude of the pooled effect is uncertain and is likely to change with new studies.

Very low: One cannot be certain about the effects of the intervention.

One of the difficulties in using GRADE is that the evidence base for an outcome may include studies with varying methodological quality and sample size. Therefore, the weight of the studies in the estimation of the pooled effect was included to make judgments about the quality of the set of included studies. The criteria used to grade the quality of evidence are shown in **Table I**. The following briefly describes how these criteria were used:

Study design

The included studies were classified as:

1. RCTs –including RCTs or cluster-RCTs
2. non-randomized experimental studies

3. observational studies, including cohort studies and case-control studies (studies with other observational designs were not included)

If a majority of evidence was from RCTs, indicated by over 50% weight in the pooled effect, a score of 0 was given. A score of -0.5 was given if a majority of evidence was from non-randomized experimental studies, and -1.0 if the evidence was from observational studies.

Limitations in methods

Four criteria were used for assessing limitations in the methods of included studies. A set of studies could receive a maximum of -2.0 points for limitations in methods.

1. *Risk of selection bias:* Appropriate allocation concealment and RCT design almost rule out this bias. Allocation is considered to be concealed if (i) central allocation is used including telephone, web-based and pharmacy-controlled randomization; (ii) sequentially numbered intervention packaging of identical appearance; (iii) study reported to be double-blind, placebo-controlled trial; or (iv) sequentially-numbered, opaque, sealed envelopes used.

   If a majority of evidence was from RCTs that reported adequate allocation concealment, a score of 0 was given. If allocation concealment was not done or was unclear in a majority of studies, a score of -0.5 was given. On reviewing the methods used in cohort or case-control studies, if the groups (exposed/unexposed in cohort studies, or cases/controls in case-control studies) were likely to be comparable at baseline and there was a low risk of reverse causality, a score of 0 was given; otherwise, the study was graded-0.5).

2. *Risk of measurement bias:* Measurement bias can be minimized by blinding the participants and researchers to the intervention. If that is not possible, the observers measuring outcome can be blinded. Lastly, measurement bias is less likely if the outcome is "objective". If the majority of evidence was from studies where any of the above was done, a score of 0 was given (otherwise, the study was graded-0.5).

3. *Loss to follow-up:* A large loss to follow-up can lead to bias in results; 20% loss to follow-up was chosen arbitrarily as the cut-off point. If the majority of evidence was from studies where loss to follow-up was less than 20%, a score of 0 was given (otherwise, 0.5 was given).

4. *Appropriateness of analysis:* If the majority of evidence was from RCTs which had analysis by intention to treat, and additionally cluster adjustment was done when the design was cluster-RCT, a score of 0 was given (otherwise, -0.5 was given). If the majority of evidence was from observational studies with analysis adjusted for confounding, a score of 0 was given (otherwise, -0.5 was given).

Precision

Results are imprecise when studies include relatively few patients and few events and thus have wide CIs around the estimate of the effect. In this case, the quality of the evidence is lower than it otherwise would be due to resulting uncertainty in the results.

If the 95% CI around the pooled effect **included no effect,** and the upper or lower confidence limits *do not* include an effect that, if real, would represent a meaningful benefit or an unacceptable harm, a score of 0 was given. Otherwise, a score of -1.0 was given.

If the 95% CI around the pooled effect **excluded no effect,** and <u>both</u> the upper or lower confidence limits are an effect that, if real, would represent a meaningful benefit or an unacceptable harm, a score of 0 was given. Otherwise, a score of -0.5 was given.

Meaningful benefit or unacceptable harm: For the purposes of these guidelines, a RR of 0.9 or lower, or a MD greater than 0.1 standard deviation (SD) was used as a guide for meaningful benefit. This translated to 10% or greater relative reduction in mortality, 10% or greater relative reduction in severe morbidity, MD higher by 1 point in mental development scores, and MD in weight higher by 100 g and length by 0.3 cm (the last at 6-18 months of age). Similarly, unacceptable harm involved a 10% or greater increase in mortality or morbidity, at least 1 point lower mean mental development score, 100 g lower weight and 0.3 cm lower length.

Consistency

Consistency refers to the similarity of estimates of effect across studies. If three or more studies were available, effect size was such that it indicated meaningful benefit or unacceptable harm, and ≥75% of evidence from at least two studies have effect sizes in the same direction as the pooled effect, a score of 0 was given. If the pooled effect size excluded meaningful benefit or unacceptable harm, and the effect size of studies with ≥75% of the total weight of evidence also excluded meaningful benefit and unacceptable harm (i.e. consistent with "no effect"), a score of 0 was also given. If the two above conditions were not satisfied, a score of -1.0 was given.

If only two studies were available, and the results were in the same direction, we gave a score of -0.5. However, if the results of the two studies were in different directions, a score of -1.0 was given. In case only one study was available, a score of -1.0 was given.

Directness

Directness, generalizability, external validity of study results or their applicability were used as synonymous. If the majority of evidence was from studies with both population and intervention the same as the population and intervention of interest, a score of 0 was given. If the majority of evidence was from studies that had a population and intervention that were different from the population or intervention of interest for these guidelines, a score of -1.0 was given; if either of them were different a score of -0.5 was given.

Upgrading quality of evidence from observational studies

The GRADE criteria were modified to start with a score of -1.0 (moderate quality) for observational studies rather than the usual -2.0 (low quality). Therefore, the quality of evidence from observational studies was not upgraded even if the effect sizes were large, there was a dose-response gradient or the confounding factors could only underestimate the true size of effect. However, the quality of evidence from observational studies was downgraded if there were serious limitations in methods, imprecision, inconsistency and indirectness as described above.

Formulation of recommendations

The external guideline panel formulated the first version of the recommendations based on the technical review published in 2006. This version of guidelines was field tested in health facilities in four countries - Ghana, India, Pakistan and Uganda - in 2008-9.

After the evidence base was updated in 2010 and its quality graded using the modified GRADE approach, WHO staff prepared the second version of recommendations in a format consistent with the new WHO *Handbook for Guideline Development*[1]. This version was sent to the external expert panel for their review and inputs, which was incorporated into the final version of the guidelines.

The GRADE system for grading recommendations was used. The strength of a recommendation reflects the degree of confidence that the desirable effects of adherence to a recommendation outweigh the undesirable effects. The decisions were made on the basis of evidence of benefits and harms, quality of evidence, values and preferences of policy-makers, health-care providers and parents, and whether costs are qualitatively justifiable compared to the benefits in low- and middle-income countries. The recommendations were graded as one of three types:

A ***strong recommendation*** is one for which there is confidence that the benefits either clearly outweigh the harms or do not. The quality of evidence required to make such a recommendation is at least moderate, although the panel may make exceptions. Similarly, the benefits are likely to be valued highly, and costs appear to be justified by the benefits of making such a recommendation. A strong recommendation can be in favor of an intervention or against it.

A ***weak recommendation*** is one for which the benefits probably outweigh the harms, but there is high quality evidence; uncertainty in how policy-makers, health workers and parents value the example, some recommendations were considered relevant only to settings in low- and middle- others were considered relevant only to settings where certain facilities were available (e.g. Recommendations 2 and 17).

---

[1] WHO. *Handbook for guideline development.* Geneva, WHO, 2008.

Table I. Modified GRADE criteria for assessing quality of evidence

Design	Limitations in methods				Precision	Consistency	Directness	Overall quality of evidence
	Based on methods of studies with ≥50% of weight of evidence							
Based on design of studies with ≥50% of weight of evidence	**Allocation concealment** (*the two groups comparable and low risk of reverse causality*)	**Blinding or other approaches to reduce measurement bias**	**Loss to follow-up**	**Analysis intention to treat; cluster adjusted if applicable** (*adjusted for confounding*)	Based on 95% CI of the pooled effect size	Based on the direction of effect size of ≥2 studies with ≥75% of weight of evidence	Based on directness of studies with ≥50% of weight of evidence	Based on the total of score in columns on the left
If RCT, then = 0 If quasi-RCT, then = -0.5 (*If observational, then = -1.0*)	If allocation concealment adequate, then = 0 If allocation concealment inadequate/unknown, then = -0.5 Not applicable if quasi-randomized 0.5 (*If observational studies adjusted for confounding, then = 0; if not, then = -0.5*)	If blinding of intervention, then = 0 If "objective" outcome, then = 0 If outcome not "objective" but observers blinded, then = 0; if not, then = -0.5 If representative cross sectional surveys, then = 0; if not, then = -0.5 If difference in measurement procedures for the two comparison groups, then = -0.5	If cohort followed up, and <20% lost, if not, then = 0.5	If intent to treat analysis, then = 0; if not, then = -0.5 If cluster RCT and analysis cluster-adjusted, then = 0; if not, then = 0 (*If observation-al studies adjusted for confounding, then = 0, if not, then = -0.5*)	If CI does not include "null", and both CI limits indicate meaningful benefit or unacceptable harm, then = 0 If CI does not include "null", but CI wider than above, then = -0.5 If CI includes "null", and both CI limits exclude meaningful benefit or unacceptable harm, then = 0 If CI includes "null", but CI limits indicate no effect, then = 0 If CI includes "null", but CI wider than as above, then = -1.0	If ≥3 studies and pooled effect indicates meaningful benefit or unacceptable harm, and individual studies in the same direction as pooled effect, then = 0, if not, then = -1.0 If ≥3 studies and pooled effect indicates no effect, and individual studies also indicate no effect, then = 0, if not, then = -1.0 If only 2 studies with ESs in same direction or both ESs consistent with no effect, then = 0.5, if ESs in different directions, then = -1.0 If single study, then = 1.0	If population as well as intervention in studies same as those of interest, then = 0 If one of the two different from that of interest, then = -0.5 If both different from those of interest, then = -1.0	If final score = 0 or -0.5, then **HIGH** If final score = -1 or -1.5, then **MODERATE** If final score = -2 or -2.5, then **LOW** If final score ≤-3, then **VERY LOW**

RECOMMENDATIONS

WHAT MILK SHOULD LBW INFANTS BE FED?

QUESTION 1: In LBW infants (P), what is the effect of feeding ***mother's own milk*** (I) compared with feeding infant formula (C) on mortality, severe morbidity, neurodevelopment and anthropometric status (O)?

Summary of evidence: No RCTs examining the effect of feeding mother's own milk to LBW infants on their mortality were identified. Therefore, evidence was considered from four observational studies, all from developed country settings. The quality of evidence for this outcome was graded as low. The pooled effect was 18% reduction in mortality (95% CI 7% to 28%).

Only two RCTs conducted in a developing country examined the effect of feeding mother's own milk on the risk of severe infections or necrotizing enterocolitis (NEC). Therefore, their results were pooled with those of six observational studies from developed country settings. The quality of evidence for this outcome was graded as moderate. The pooled effect was 60% reduction (95% CI 48% to 69%) in the risk of severe infections or NEC.

Eight observational studies evaluated the effect of feeding mother's own milk on neurodevelopment. The outcome in six of these studies was the MD in mental development scores between breast-milk-fed and formula-fed LBW infants at different ages ranging from 18 months to 8 years. The quality of evidence for this outcome was graded as low. The pooled MD in mental development scores was 5.2 points higher (95% CI 3.6 to 6.8) in those fed mother's own milk. Two studies could not be included in the meta-analysis. One of them reported higher mental development scores at 6 months of age in breast-milk-fed infants but did not report CIs of this difference (MD 10 points). The other study reported adjusted OR for higher- than-average scores in an English picture vocabulary test at 5 years of age (OR 1.06, 95% CI 0.86 to 1.32).

Only one observational study reported the effect of feeding mother's own milk on anthropometric status at 9 months of age. The quality of evidence for this outcome was graded as very low. This study found no significant difference in weight SD scores (MD -0.27, 95% CI -0.59 to 0.05) but significantly lower length SD scores in infants fed mother's own milk compared with formula (MD -0.47, 95% CI -0.79 to -0.15).

Long-term beneficial effects of breast-milk feeding on blood pressure, serum lipid profile and pro-insulin levels have also been reported; these studies were not reviewed in detail.

In conclusion, there is low to moderate quality evidence that feeding mother's own milk to LBW infants of any gestation is associated with lower mortality, lower incidence of infections and NEC, and improved development scores as compared with feeding infant formula. There is very low quality evidence that feeding mother's own milk is associated with lower length at 9 months of age. (See GRADE profile, **Table 1**).

Balance of benefits and harms, values and preferences, and costs: Important benefits were found for mortality (18% reduction), severe infections or NEC (60% reduction), and mental development scores (5.2 points higher) associated with feeding mother's own milk compared with formula. The only apparent harm was lower length at 9 months in one study.

Policy-makers, health-care providers and parents in low- and middle-countries are likely to give a high value to the benefits in reduced mortality and severe morbidity. Benefits in terms of increased mental development scores would be valued in both developed and low- and middle-income countries.

Considering the low costs involved in implementation of feeding mother's own milk, the observed benefits are clearly worth the costs.

RECOMMENDATION 1

LBW infants, including those with VLBW, should be fed mother's own milk.

(Strong recommendation, based on moderate quality evidence of reduced severe morbidity and low quality evidence of reduced mortality and improved neurodevelopment)

Table 1. GRADE profile summary for Question 1[1-21]

(see annexes for detailed GRADE profiles and summary tables of individual studies)

OUTCOME	No. of studies	Design	Limitations in methods (comparabil-ity of groups, measure-ment of outcomes or analysis)	Precision	Consistency	General-izability/ direct-ness	Overall quality of evidence	Pooled effect size (95% CI) or range of effect sizes if pooling not possible at all
Mortality (to discharge in 1 study, to neonatal period in 2 studies, post neonatal in 1 study)	4	All observati on-al studies (-1.0)	No serious limitations (0)	Pooled effect significant, but upper limit of CI close to null (-0.5)	ES of 3 studies with >75% of total weight in the same direction as pooled effect (0)	Majority of evidence from studies in developed countries (-0.5)	**LOW** (Total -2.0)	OR 0.82 (0.72 to 0.93)
Severe infection or NEC (until discharge)	8	Majority of evidence from observati on-al studies (-1.0)	No serious limitations (0)	Pooled effect significant and upper limit of CI is meaningful (0)	All studies in same direction (0)	Majority of evidence from studies in developed countries (-0.5)	**MODER-ATE** (Total -0.5)	OR 0.40 (0.31 to 0.52)
Neuro-developme nt (Mental development score at 18 months to 8 years)	6	All observati on-al studies (-1.0)	Limitations in outcome measurement (-0.5)	Pooled effect significant and lower limit of CI meaningful (0)	ES of studies with >75% of total weight in the same direction as pooled effect (0)	Majority of evidence from studies in developed countries (-0.5)	**LOW** (Total -2.0)	MD 5.2 points (3.6, 6.8)
Anthropo-metric status (weight and length SD scores at 9 months)	1	All observati on-al studies (-1.0)	Limitations in analysis (-0.5)	Pooled effect not significant for weight; significant for length, but upper limit of CI close to null (-0.5)	Single study (-1.0)	Study from developed country setting (-0.5)	**VERY LOW** (Total -3.5)	MD in: weight SD score -0.27 (-0.59, 0.05) length SD score -0.47 (-0.79, -0.15)

QUESTION 2: In LBW infants who cannot be fed mother's own milk (P), what is the effect of feeding *donor human milk* (I) compared with feeding infant formula (C) on mortality, severe morbidity, neurodevelopment and anthropometric status (O)?

Summary of evidence: All studies included in the evidence base for this question were RCTs. All had very few methodological limitations and most were conducted in developed country settings.

Evidence from 3 RCTs showed that there was no significant effect of feeding donor human milk compared with feeding infant formula on mortality (RR 0.81, 95% CI 0.46, 1.41). The evidence was judged to be of moderate quality largely because of the wide CI of effect which reflects lack of sufficient data for this outcome.

The pooled effect in five RCTs and one non-randomized experimental study was 61% reduction (95% CI 22% to 81%) in the risk of severe infections or NEC when LBW infants were fed donor human milk compared with feeding infant formula. The quality of evidence for this outcome was graded as high.

A multi-centre RCT conducted in the United States of America compared the effects of an exclusively human milk-based diet compared with a diet of both human milk and bovine milk-based products in infants with birth weight from 500 g to 1250 g. The intervention groups received mother's own milk (or donor human milk if mother's own milk was not available) with a human milk-based human-milk fortifier, while the control group received mother's own milk (or formula if mother's own milk was not available) with bovine milk-based human-milk fortifier. This study was not included in the GRADE profile (**Table 2**) because both groups received mother's own milk, if it was available. The study reported a 77% reduction (95% CI 34% to 92%) in the odds of developing NEC in the group that received an exclusive human-milk diet.

Only two RCTs have examined the effect of feeding donor human milk compared with feeding infant formula on mental development scores. There was no significant difference in scores (MD in scores -1.2 points, 95% CI -5.1 to 2.6) between the intervention and comparison groups. The quality of evidence for this outcome was low.

Similarly, only two RCTs were identified that examined the effect of donor human milk on anthropometric status at 18 months of age. There was no significant difference in weight (MD -0.1 kg, 95% CI -0.35 to 0.15) or length (MD -0.53 cm, 95% CI -1.2 to 0.14 cm) between infants fed donor human milk or infant formula. The quality of this evidence is low.

In conclusion, there is high quality evidence that feeding donor human milk to LBW infants is associated with lower incidence of infections and NEC during the initial hospital stay after birth. There is moderate quality evidence for no significant effect on mortality, and low quality evidence of no effect on mental development scores and anthropometric status at 18 months of age.

Balance of benefits and harms, values and preferences, and costs: Important benefits were found for severe infections or NEC (61% reduction). There was no significant effect on mortality, neurodevelopment or anthropometric status (see GRADE profile, **Table 2**). The risks are related to transmission of infections, such as human immunodeficiency virus (HIV), in case safe milk-banking facilities are not available.

Given the high mortality in low- and middle-income country populations, particularly as a result of infections, the benefit in terms of reduction of severe infections or NEC would be highly valued by policy-makers, health-care providers and parents in these settings.

The observed benefits would be considered to be worth the costs in many settings. However, the necessity of safe milk-banking facilities for feeding of donor human milk to reduce the risk of HIV and other infections could make the costs of this intervention unaffordable in very resource-limited settings.

- ▪ **RECOMMENDATION 2**

LBW infants, including those with VLBW, who cannot be fed mother's own milk should be fed donor human milk.

(Strong situational recommendation relevant to settings where safe and affordable milk-banking facilities are available or can be set up, based on high quality evidence for benefit in reducing severe morbidity)

Table 2. GRADE profile summary for Question 2[22-27]

(see annexes for detailed GRADE profiles and summary tables of individual studies)

OUTCOME	No. of studies	Design	Limitations in methods (comparability of groups, measurement of outcomes or analysis)	Precision	Consistency	General-izability/ directness	Overall quality of evidence	Pooled effect size (95% CI) or range of effect sizes if pooling not possible at all
Mortality (until discharge in 1 study, until 9 months in the other 2 studies)	3	All RCTs (0)	No serious limitations (0)	Pooled effect not significant, with wide CI (-1.0)	ES of two studies with >75% of total weight in the same direction as the pooled effect (0)	All studies from developed country settings (-0.5)	**MODERATE** (Total -1.5)	RR 0.81 (0.46, 1.41)
Severe infection or NEC (until discharge)	6	Most evidence from RCTs (0)	No serious limitations (0)	Pooled effect significant, upper limit of CI indicates meaningful effect (0)	ES of all studies in the same direction as the pooled effect (0)	Most evidence from studies in developed country settings (-0.5)	**HIGH** (Total -0.5)	RR 0.39 (0.19, 0.78)
Neuro-development (mental development score at 18 months)	2	Both RCTs (0)	No serious limitations (0)	Pooled effect not significant, with wide CI (-1.0)	Only two studies, ES of both in same direction (-0.5)	Both studies from developed country settings (-0.5)	**LOW** (Total -2.0)	MD -1.2 points (-5.1, 2.6)
Anthropo-metric status (weight and length at 18 months)	2	Both RCTs (0)	No serious limitations (0)	Pooled effect not significant, with wide CI (-1.0)	Only two studies, ES of both consistent with no effect (-0.5)	Both studies from developed country settings (-0.5)	**LOW** (Total -2.0)	MD in: weight -0.1 kg (-0.35, 0.15) length -0.53 cm (-1.2, 0.14)

QUESTION 3: In LBW infants who cannot be fed mother's own milk or donor human milk (P), what is the effect of feeding ***preterm infant formula*** (I) compared with feeding standard infant formula (C) on mortality, severe morbidity, neurodevelopment and anthropometric status (O)?

Summary of evidence: Only one RCT each reporting the effect of preterm infant formula compared with that of standard infant formula on mortality, neurodevelopment and anthropometric status was identified. The quality of evidence for all outcomes was low. No studies examined the effect of the intervention on severe morbidity. There was no significant effect on mortality up to 18 months of age (RR 1.1, 95% CI 0.72 to 1.69), Intelligence quotient (IQ) scores at 8 years of age (MD 4.8 points, 95% CI -0.6 to 10.2) or anthropometric status at 18 months of age (MD in weight 0.2 kg, 95% CI -0.32 to 0.72; MD in length 1.2 cm, 95% CI -0.28 to 2.68). Short-term weight gain was higher in infants fed preterm infant formula than in those fed standard infant formula (13 g versus 16 g/kg per day). (See GRADE profile, **Table 3**).

Balance of benefits and harms, values and preferences, and costs: There was no significant difference in any critical outcome. However, confidence in this finding of equivalence is low given the low quality of evidence and wide CIs of all results. The cost of preterm infant formula is high, its availability in resource-limited settings is low, and evidence of benefits is unclear.

- ### RECOMMENDATION 3

LBW infants, including those with VLBW, who cannot be fed mother's own milk or donor human milk should be fed standard infant formula.

(Weak situational recommendation relevant for resource-limited settings, based on evidence of no significant benefit of preterm infant formula on mortality, neurodevelopment and long-term growth)

VLBW infants who cannot be fed mother's own milk or donor human milk should be given preterm infant formula if they fail to gain weight despite adequate feeding with standard infant formula.

(Weak situational recommendation relevant for resource-limited settings, based on benefit of preterm formula on short-term growth)

Table 3. GRADE profile summary for Question 3[28-30]

(see annexes for detailed GRADE profiles and summary tables of individual studies)

OUTCOME	No. of studies	Design	Limitations in methods	Precision	Consistency	General-izability/ directness	Overall quality of evidence	Pooled effect size (95% CI) or range of effect sizes if pooling not possible at all
Mortality (up to 18 months of age)	1	RCT (0)	No serious limitations (0)	Not significant, with wide CI (-1.0)	Single study (-1.0)	From high-income setting (-0.5)	**LOW** (Total - 2.5)	RR 1.1 (0.72 to 1.69)
Neuro-development (IQ scores at 8 years of age)	1	RCT (0)	No serious limitations (0)	Not significant, with wide CI (-1.0)	Single study (-1.0)	From high-income setting (-0.5)	**LOW** (Total - 2.5)	MD 4.8 points (-0.6 to 10.2)
Anthropo-metric status (at 18 months of age)	1	RCT (0)	No serious limitations (0)	Not significant, with wide CI (-1.0)	Single study (-1.0)	From high-income setting (-0.5)	**LOW** (Total - 2.5)	MD in: weight 0.2 kg (-0.32, 0.72) length 1.2 cm (-0.28, 2.68)

QUESTION 4: In LBW infants who cannot be fed mother's own milk or donor human milk (P), what is the effect of feeding *nutrient-enriched infant formula* from hospital discharge until 6 months of age (I) compared with feeding standard infant formula (C) on mortality, severe morbidity, neurodevelopment and anthropometric status (O)?

Summary of evidence: No studies were found which examined the effect of the intervention on mortality or severe morbidity. Two RCTs were identified which reported the effect of nutrient-enriched infant formula compared with that of standard infant formula on neurodevelopment. The quality of evidence was low. Five RCTs examined the effect of the intervention on anthropometric status at 12 to 18 months of age. The quality of evidence for this outcome was graded as low. There was no significant effect on mental development scores (MD 0.2 points, 95% CI -3.0 to 3.4) or weight (MD 0.1 kg, 95% CI -0.3 to 0.4) and length at 18 months of age (MD 0.5 cm, 95% CI -0.5 to 1.4). (See GRADE profile, **Table 4.**)

Balance of benefits and harms, values and preferences, and costs: There was no significant effect on neurodevelopment or anthropometric status at 12 to 18 months of age. The cost of nutrient-enriched infant formula is high and its availability in resource-limited settings is low. The observed lack of benefits does not justify the costs in such settings.

- ■ **RECOMMENDATION 4**

LBW infants, including those with VLBW, who cannot be fed mother's own milk or donor human milk should be fed standard infant formula from the time of discharge until 6 months of age.

(Weak situational recommendation relevant for resource-limited settings, based on low quality evidence for no benefit of nutrient-enriched formula on critical outcomes)

Table 4. GRADE profile summary for Question 4[21, 31-34]

(see annexes for detailed GRADE tables and summary tables of individual studies)

OUTCOME	No. of studies	Design	Limitations in methods	Precision	Consistency	General-izability/ directness	Overall quality of evidence	Pooled effect size (95% CI) or range of effect sizes if pooling not possible at all
Neuro-developme nt (mental development scores at 18 months)	2	RCTs (0)	No serious limitations (0)	Pooled effect not significant, with wide CI (-1.0)	Only two studies, ES of both consistent with no effect (-0.5)	Both studies from developed country settings (-0.5)	**LOW** (Total -2.0)	MD 0.2 points (-3.0, 3.4)
Anthropo-metric status (at 12-18 months of age)	5	RCTs (0)	No serious limitations (0)	Pooled effect not significant, with wide CI (1.0)	Pooled effect size indicates no effect, ES of studies with <75% weight consistent with no effect (-1.0)	All studies from developed country settings (-0.5)	**LOW** (Total -2.5)	MD in: weight 0.1 kg (-0.3, 0.4) length 0.5 cm (-0.5, 1.4)

QUESTION 5: In VLBW infants who are fed mother's own milk or donor human milk (P), what is the effect of ***multi-component fortification*** of breast milk (I) compared with no fortification of breast milk (C) on mortality, severe morbidity, neurodevelopment and anthropometric status (O)?

Summary of evidence: Two studies reported the impact of multi-component fortification on mortality rates in VLBW infants. The quality of evidence for this outcome was graded as low. There was no significant difference in the risk of mortality between infants who received human milk fortification and those who did not receive fortified milk (pooled RR 2.32, 95% CI 0.16 to 34.7).

A total of six studies, four RCTs from developed country settings and two quasi-RCTs from developing country settings, have evaluated the effect of human milk fortification on the risk of NEC in preterm neonates. The quality of evidence for this outcome was graded as very low. No significant difference in the risk of NEC was observed between the groups supplemented with a multi-component fortifier and the control groups (pooled RR 1.22, 95% CI 0.6 to 2.46).

A multi-centre RCT conducted in the United States of America compared the effects of an exclusively human milk-based diet compared with a diet of both human milk and bovine milk-based products in infants with birth weights of 500 g to 1250 g. The intervention groups received mother's own milk (or donor human milk if mother's own milk was not available) with a human milk-based human-milk fortifier, while the control group received mother's own milk (or formula if mother's own milk was not available) with bovine milk-based human-milk fortifier. This study was not included in the GRADE profile (**Table 5**) because both groups received a fortifier. The study reported a 77% reduction (95% CI 34% to 92%) in the odds of developing NEC in the group that received an exclusive human-milk diet (including human milk-based fortifier)

Only one RCT which examined the effect of multi-component fortification on long-term neurodevelopmental outcomes was identified. The study did not find any significant difference in mental development scores at 18 months of age between the fortified and unfortified groups of infants (MD 2.2 points, 95% CI -3.3 to 7.7). The quality of evidence was low.

Two RCTs looked at the impact of fortification of human milk on anthropometric status at 6 months of age or older. No significant effect was observed in either the weight (pooled MD -0.03 kg, 95% CI -0.32 to 0.25 kg) or length (pooled MD -0.2 cm, 95% CI -1.0 to 0.6) at 12 to 18 months of age in infants who received fortified human milk during the neonatal period. The quality of evidence for this outcome was graded as low.

Evidence was also examined for a non-critical outcome – short-term growth during initial hospital stay. Nine RCTs examined the effect of multi-component fortification of human milk on the rate of weight gain. The quality of evidence was graded as moderate. The pooled result was that weight gain was 2.75 g/kg per day (95% CI 1.6 to 3.9) greater in infants receiving human-milk fortifier. Similarly, the pooled effect on rate of length gain was 0.18 cm per week (95% CI 0.09 to 0.28) greater than the control group.

In conclusion, there is low to very low quality evidence that feeding multi-component fortified human milk does not affect the risk of mortality and NEC, and does not improve neurodevelopmental outcomes and anthropometric status at 6 months of age or beyond. Human-milk fortifier improves the rates of weight and length gain during the initial hospital stay (see GRADE profile, **Table 5**).

Balance of benefits and harms, values and preferences, and costs: There was no evidence of significant benefits or harm in mortality, NEC, mental development scores, and anthropometric status associated with feeding fortified human milk. However, the possibility of harm in terms of increased risk of mortality and NEC cannot be entirely ruled out, because the point estimates were above 1 but with very wide CIs. The only benefit observed was in short-term growth during initial hospital stay.

Given the evidence of lack of benefits in any of the critical outcomes and a substantial improvement in weight gain during hospital stay, it is likely that clinicians would value this intervention but policy-makers would not. The costs are significant and may not be justified in resource-limited settings by the small observed benefits. Also, the availability of multi-component fortifier might be an issue in many such settings.

- ## RECOMMENDATION 5

VLBW infants who are fed mother's own milk or donor human milk need not be given bovine milk-based human-milk fortifier. VLBW infants who fail to gain weight despite adequate breast-milk feeding should be given human-milk fortifiers, preferably those that are human milk based.

(Weak situational recommendation relevant to resource-limited settings, based on low to very low quality evidence for no benefits in critical outcomes and higher costs)

Table 6. GRADE profile summary for Question 5[27, 35-46]

(see annexes for detailed GRADE profiles and summary tables of individual studies)

OUTCOME	No. of studies	Design	Limitations in methods	Precision	Consistency	General-izability/ directness	Overall quality of evidence	Pooled effect size (95% CI) or range of effect sizes if pooling not possible at all
Mortality (until discharge in 1 study, until 3 months of age in other study)	2	Majority of evidence from RCTs (0)	No serious limitations (0)	Pooled effect not significant, with wide CI (-1.0)	Only two studies, effect in different directions (-1.0)	Majority of evidence from the study in developed country settings (-0.5)	**LOW** (Total -2.5)	RR 2.32 (0.16, 34.7)
Severe morbidity (NEC until discharge)	6	Most evidence from RCTs (0)	Limitations in measurement and analysis (-1.0)	Pooled effect not significant, with wide CI (-1.0)	ES of studies with <75% of total weight in the same direction as pooled ES (-1.0)	Majority of evidence from studies in developed country settings (-0.5)	**VERY LOW** (Total -3.5)	RR 1.22 (0.6, 2.46)
Neurodevelopment (mental development score at 18 months)	1	RCT (0)	No serious limitations (0)	Not significant, with wide CI (-1.0)	Single study (-1.0)	From developed country setting (-0.5)	**LOW** (Total -2.5)	MD 2.2 points (-3.3, 7.7)
Anthropometric status (at 12-18 months)	2	RCTs (0)	No serious limitations (0)	Pooled effect not significant, with wide CI (-1.0)	Only two studies, ES of both consistent with no effect (-0.5)	Both studies from developed country setting (-0.5)	**LOW** (Total -2.0)	MD in: weight -0.03 kg (-0.32, 0.25); length -0.2 cm (-1.0, 0.6)
Short-term gain in weight and length[+] (during initial hospital stay)	9 (8 RCTs, 1 quasi-RCT)	Most evidence from RCTs (0)	Limitations in follow-up and analysis (-1.0)	Pooled effect significant and lower limit of CI meaningful (0)	Studies with ≥75% of total weight in the same direction as pooled effect (0)	Majority of evidence from studies in developed country settings (-0.5)	**MODERATE** (Total -1.5)	MD in: weight gain 2.75 g/kg per day (-1.6, 3.9) length gain 0.18 cm per week (0.09, 0.28)

QUESTION 6: In VLBW infants who are fed mother's own milk or donor human milk (P), what is the effect of giving 2-4 times the recommended daily allowance (RDA) of ***vitamin D supplements*** (I) compared with 1 RDA of vitamin D supplements (C) on mortality, severe morbidity, neurodevelopment and anthropometric status (O)?

Summary of evidence: Two RCTs examined the effect of 2-4 RDA vitamin D supplementation compared with 1 RDA supplementation on anthropometric status at 6 months of age or older. While one RCT reported weight percentiles and length SD scores at 9 to 11 years, the other study reported weight and length at 6 months of age. Neither of the studies found any significant effect on anthropometric status. The quality of evidence was graded as very low.

Two RCTs evaluated the effect of 2-4 RDA vitamin D supplements on bone mineralization status of preterm neonates at 6 months of age or older. The quality of evidence was very low. There was no difference in the bone mineral densities of infants who received 2-4 RDA and 1 RDA vitamin D supplements respectively (pooled MD 2.0 mg/cm², 95% CI -8.0 to 12.0). Another study, an RCT from a developed country, ascertained the effect on radiographic bone disease at 6 weeks of age in preterm VLBW infants. The study did not find any difference in the scores (graded on a scale of 0 to 9, with 0 being normal and 9 indicating severe bone disease) between the two groups (median score 2 versus 2.5, P=0.36).

To conclude, there is very low quality evidence that giving 2-4 RDA oral vitamin D supplements does not affect anthropometric status or bone mineralization at or beyond 6 months of age in VLBW infants. (See GRADE profile, **Table 6**.)

Balance of benefits and harms, values and preferences, and costs: There is no evidence of benefits or harm associated with daily oral vitamin D supplementation in doses exceeding 1 RDA in VLBW infants. Given the evidence of lack of benefits in any of the critical outcomes, policy-makers and health-care providers from both low- and middle-income and developed countries are unlikely to give high value to high-dose vitamin D supplementation in VLBW infants. Further, availability of formulations containing only vitamin D for daily supplementation of LBW infants is low. The lack of evidence of benefit on any critical outcome does not justify the costs of making such formulations widely available.

- **RECOMMENDATION 6**

VLBW infants should be given vitamin D supplements at a dose ranging from400 i.u to 1000 i.u. per day until 6 months of age.

(Weak recommendation, based on very low quality evidence for lack of benefits)

Table 6. GRADE profile summary for Question 6[47-49]

(see annexes for detailed GRADE profiles and summary tables of individual studies)

OUTCOME	No. of studies	Design	Limitations in methods	Precision	Consistency	Generalizability/directness	Overall quality of evidence	Pooled effect size (95 % CI) or range of effect sizes if pooling not possible at all
Anthropometric status (at 9-11 years)	1	RCT (0)	Limitations in allocation of subjects, follow-up, and analysis (-1.5)	Effect not significant, with wide CI (-1.0)	Single study (-1.0)	From developed country setting (-0.5)	**VERY LOW** (Total -4.0)	MD in: weight percentiles 2.5 (-13.0, 18.0) length SD scores -0.21 (-1.4, 0.9)
Bone mineral density (at 6 months in one study, at 9-11 years in the other study)	2	RCTs (0)	Limitations in allocation of subjects and analysis (-1.0)	Pooled effect not significant, with wide CI (-1.0)	Only two studies, ES of both consistent with no effect (-0.5)	Both from developed country settings (-0.5)	**VERY LOW** (Total -3.0)	MD 2 mg/cm² (-8, 12)

QUESTION 7: In LBW infants who are fed mother's own milk or donor human milk (P), what is the effect of *calcium and phosphorus supplementation* (I) compared with no supplementation (C) on mortality, severe morbidity, neurodevelopment and anthropometric status (O)?

Summary of evidence: No studies were identified that examined the effect of calcium and phosphorus supplementation on mortality, neurodevelopment or anthropometric status in preterm VLBW infants.

Only one RCT examined the effect of calcium and/or phosphorus supplementation on rickets of prematurity in VLBW infants. Therefore, additional evidence from an observational study was considered. Both the studies were from developed country settings. The quality of evidence for this outcome was graded as very low. There was no significant difference in the incidence of rickets between the intervention and control groups (pooled RR 0.35, 95% CI 0.03 to 4.75).

One RCT looked at the effect of mineral supplementation on the risk of active metabolic bone disease (high alkaline phosphatase levels) in preterm neonates. The quality of evidence for this outcome was graded as low. The study showed a 45% reduction (95% CI 18% to 63%) in the risk of metabolic bone disease following calcium and phosphorus supplementation. Another study - a historical cohort from a developed country - evaluated the effect on the alkaline phosphatase levels in ELBW infants. The study found significantly lower levels in infants who received phosphate supplementation than in those who received neither calcium nor phosphorus supplementation (median [range]: 484 [139, phosphatase levels of infants who received both calcium and phosphate supplements were not significantly different from the group that received neither of the supplements (median [range]: 605 [166, 1453] versus 684 [168, 2220] respectively; P>0.05).

In conclusion, there is low quality evidence that routine calcium and phosphate supplementation reduces the risk of metabolic bone disease in preterm VLBW infants. There is, however, no evidence of reduction in the risk of rickets of prematurity. (See GRADE profile, **Table 7**.)

Balance of benefits and harms, values and preferences, and costs: There is lack of evidence for benefits or harm in mortality, neurodevelopment, and anthropometric status following routine calcium and phosphorus supplementation. The intervention has some benefit in reducing metabolic bone disease in preterm VLBW infants.

The benefit in terms of reducing metabolic bone disease is expected to be valued by health-care providers and parents. The associated costs are likely to be low and may be justified by the benefits.

■ **RECOMMENDATION 7**

VLBW infants who are fed mother's own milk or donor human milk should be given daily calcium (120-140 mg/kg per day) and phosphorus (60-90 mg/kg per day) supplementation during the first months of life.

(Weak recommendation, based on low quality evidence for benefit in a non-critical outcome)

Table 7. GRADE profile summary for Question 7[50-52]

(see annexes for detailed GRADE profiles and summary tables of individual studies)

OUTCOME	No. of studies	Design	Limitations in methods	Precision	Consistency	General-izability/ directness	Overall quality of evidence	Pooled effect size (95% CI) or range of effect sizes if pooling not possible at all
Rickets of prematurity (during the study period)	2 (1 RCT, 1 observa-tional)	Majority of evidence from the observa-tional study (-1.0)	Limitations in selection of subjects and analysis (-1.0)	Pooled effect not significant, with wide CI (-1.0)	Only two studies, ES of both in the same direction (-0.5)	Both from developed country settings (-0.5)	**VERY LOW** (Total -4.0)	RR 0.35 (0.03, 4.75)
Metabolic bone disease (until discharge)	1	RCT (0)	No serious limitations (0)	Effect significant and upper limit of CI <0.9 (0)	Single study (-1.0)	Study from developed country setting; intervention indirect (preterm formula with calcium/phos-phorus supplement) (-1.0)	**LOW** (Total -2.0)	RR 0.55 (0.37, 0.82)

QUESTION 8: In VLBW infants who are fed mother's own milk or donor human milk (P), what is the effect of starting *iron supplementation at 2 weeks of age* (I) compared with starting iron supplementation at 2 months of age (C) on mortality, severe morbidity, neurodevelopment and anthropometric status (O)?

Summary of evidence: One RCT examined the effect of early iron supplementation on mortality in VLBW infants. There was no difference in the risk of mortality up to 2 months of age between the group of infants that received early iron supplementation and the group that received iron at a later age (RR 0.94, 95% CI 0.14 to 6.56). The quality of evidence was graded as very low. The wide CIs further reduce the confidence in this outcome.

Three RCTs evaluated the effect of supplements on late onset sepsis. The quality of evidence for this outcome was graded as very low. There was no significant difference in the incidence of sepsis between the two groups (pooled RR 1.06, 95% CI 0.86 to 1.30).

Three RCTs examined the effect of supplements on significant anaemia up to 2 months of age. The quality of evidence for this outcome was graded as low. The pooled effect was 30% reduction (95% CI 6% to 48%) in the need for blood transfusion with early iron supplementation. The effect could be an underestimate of the true effect size because one of the included studies initiated iron at 4 weeks of age in the control group, unlike the other two that started iron at 2 months. Another study, a quasi-RCT from a developed country setting, found a significant reduction in the proportion of infants with haemoglobin levels <9 g/dl at 3 months of age (RR 0.03, 95% CI 0 to 0.44). The results of this study were not included in the meta-analysis because the definition of severe anaemia in the other studies was anaemia requiring blood transfusion.

One RCT studied the effect on both neurodevelopment and malnutrition at 5 years of age. The quality of evidence for both outcomes was graded as very low. The study did not find any difference in either the mental processing composite score (MD 3.0 points, 95% CI -2.1 to 8.1) or the risk of stunting (RR 1.06, 95% CI 0.3 to 3.5) between infants who received early iron supplementation and those who received it later.

Three RCTs examined the effect of early iron supplementation on morbidities attributed to oxidative stress, particularly chronic lung disease (CLD) and retinopathy of prematurity (ROP), in preterm VLBW infants. The quality of evidence for this outcome was graded as low. There was a trend towards reduction in the risk of CLD in infants who received iron at an earlier age (pooled RR 0.61, 95% CI 0.37 to 1.0). No significant difference was found in the risk of ROP (pooled RR 0.41, 95% CI 0.14 to 1.18).

To conclude, there is low quality evidence that early iron supplementation reduces severe anaemia, defined as anaemia needing blood transfusion, in early infancy, and no evidence that it improves other critical outcomes. There is low to very low quality evidence that supplementing iron does not increase the risk of severe morbidities such as late onset sepsis, CLD and ROP. (See GRADE profile, **Table 8.**)

Balance of benefits and harms, values and preferences, and costs: There is benefit in terms of reduced risk of severe anaemia and no apparent harms associated with early iron supplementation of VLBW infants. Given the evidence for lack of harmful effects, policy-makers and health-care providers in both low- and middle-income and developed country settings are likely to give a high value to the intervention. The benefits observed with iron supplementation justify the marginal costs involved in administering early iron supplements to VLBW infants.

- **RECOMMENDATION 8**

VLBW infants fed mother's own milk or donor human milk should be given 2-4 mg/kg per day iron supplementation starting at 2 weeks

(Weak recommendation, based on low quality evidence for benefit in one critical outcome and low to very low quality evidence for no harms in other critical outcomes

Table 8. GRADE profile summary for Question 8[53-57]

(see annexes for detailed GRADE profiles and summary tables of individual studies)

OUTCOME	No. of studies	Design	Limitations in methods	Precision	Consistency	General-izability / directness	Overall quality of evidence	Pooled effect size (95% CI) *or range of effect sizes if pooling not possible at all*
Mortality (until 60 days of age)	1	RCT (0)	Limitations in allocation of subjects (-0.5)	Effect not significant, with wide CI (-1.0)	Single study (-1.0)	From developed country setting (-0.5)	**VERY LOW** (Total -3.0)	RR 0.94 (0.14, 6.56)
Severe morbidity - Late onset sepsis	3	RCTs (0)	Limitations in allocation of subjects (-0.5)	Pooled effect not significant, with wide CI (-1.0)	Pooled ES indicates no effect, but ES of only one study consistent with no effect (-1.0)	Most evidence from studies in developed country settings (-0.5)	**VERY LOW** (Total -3.0)	RR 1.06 (0.86, 1.30)
Significant anaemia requiring blood transfusion (up to 2 months of age)	3	RCTs (0)	Limitations in allocation of subjects, measurement and follow-up (-1.5)	Pooled effect significant, but upper limit of CI close to null (-0.5)	ES of all studies in the same direction as pooled ES (0)	Most evidence from studies in developed country settings (-0.5)	**LOW** (Total -2.5)	RR 0.70 (0.52, 0.94)
Neurodevel opment (Mental processing composite at 5 years of age)	1	RCT (0)	Limitations in allocation of subjects and follow-up (-1.0)	Effect size not significant, with wide CI (-1.0)	Single study (-1.0)	From developed country setting (-0.5)	**VERY LOW** (Total -3.5)	MD 3.0 points (-2.1, 8.1)
Anthropom etric status (at 5 years of age)	1	RCT (0)	Limitations in allocation of subjects and follow-up (-1.0)	Effect not significant, with wide CI (-1.0)	Single study (-1.0)	From developed country setting (-0.5)	**VERY LOW** (Total -3.5)	RR for under nutrition 0.68 (0.37, 1.26) stunting 1.06 (0.3, 3.5)
CLD and ROP(during the study perio)	3	RCTs (0)	Limitations in allocation of subjects (-0.5)	Pooled effect not significant, with wide CI (-1.0)	ES of studies with ≥75% of total weight in same direction as pooled ES (0)	Most evidence from studies in developed country settings (-0.5)	**LOW** (Total -2.0)	RR for CLD 0.61 (0.37, 1.0) ROP0.41 (0.14, 1.18)

QUESTION 9: In VLBW infants who are fed mother's own milk or donor human milk (P), what is the effect of ***daily oral vitamin A supplementation*** (I) compared with no supplementation (C) on mortality, severe morbidity, neurodevelopment and anthropometric status (O)?

Summary of evidence: A Cochrane review assessed the benefits and risks of vitamin A supplementation in VLBW infants. The meta-analysis of the eight eligible trials suggested a beneficial effect in reducing death or oxygen requirement at 1 month of age (RR 0.93, 95% CI 0.88 to 0.99) and oxygen requirement at 36 weeks postmenstrual age (RR 0.87, 95% CI 0.77 to 0.98). However, of the eight studies, only one trial used the oral route for vitamin A supplementation. This study did not find any significant effect on either mortality until discharge (RR 0.86, 95% CI 0.56 to 1.33) or chronic lung disease (RR 1.0, 95% CI 0.8 to 1.24) following daily oral vitamin A supplements of 5000 i.u./kg in ELBW infants. The quality of evidence for both the outcomes was graded as low. (See GRADE profile, **Table 9**).

To conclude, daily oral vitamin A supplementation at 2-3 times the RDA does not reduce the risk of mortality or CLD in VLBW infants. However, there is insufficient evidence (a single study) to have confidence in this conclusion.

Balance of benefits and harms, values and preferences, and costs: There is low quality evidence for no benefits or harm in any of the critical outcomes with daily oral vitamin A supplementation.

Given the lack of benefits and the additional costs involved in administering daily vitamin A supplements, policy-makers and health-care providers are not likely to give high value to routine oral vitamin A supplementation in VLBW infants.

- **RECOMMENDATION 9**

Daily oral vitamin A supplementation for LBW infants who are fed mother's own milk or donor human milk is not recommended at the present time because there is not enough evidence of benefits to support such a recommendation.

(Weak recommendation, based on low quality evidence for lack of benefits in critical outcomes)

Table 9. GRADE profile summary for Question 9[58, 59]

(see annexes for detailed GRADE profiles and summary tables of individual studies)

OUTCOME	No. of studies	Design	Limitations in methods	Precision	Consistency	Generaliz ability/ directness	Overall quality of evidence	Pooled effect size (95% CI) or range of effect sizes if pooling not possible at all
Mortality (until discharge)	1	RCT	No serious limitations	Effect not significant, with wide CI	Single study	From developed country setting	**LOW**	RR 0.86 (0.56, 1.33)
		(0)	(0)	(-1.0)	(-1.0)	(-0.5)	(Total -2.5)	
Severe morbidity – CLD (at 36 weeks postmenstrua l age)	1	RCT	No serious limitations	Effect not significant, with wide CI	Single study	From developed country setting	**LOW**	RR 1.0 (0.80, 1.24)
		(0)	(0)	(-1.0)	(-1.0)	(-0.5)	(Total -2.5)	

QUESTION 10: In LBW infants who are fed mother's own milk or donor human milk (P), what is the effect of **zinc supplementation** (I) compared with no supplementation (C) on mortality, severe morbidity, neurodevelopment and anthropometric status (O)?

Summary of evidence: Two RCTs from developed country settings examined the effect of zinc supplementation on mortality in term LBW infants. The quality of evidence for this outcome was graded as low. There was no significant difference in the risk of mortality between the zinc- supplemented and the control groups (pooled OR 0.95, 95% CI 0.52 to 1.74). Another study, a community-based RCT from a developing country setting, studied the impact of zinc supplementation on mortality in term SGA infants. Only 57% of the infants were LBW and hence the results were not included in the meta-analysis. This study found a significant reduction in the risk of mortality in term SGA infants (RR 0.32, Three RCTs conducted in low- and middle-income country settings examined the effect of zinc supplementation on diarrhoeal illness during infancy. The quality of evidence for this outcome was graded as low. No significant reduction was found in the risk of diarrhoeal episodes in the first 6-12 months of life (pooled RR 0.94, 95% CI 0.82 to 1.07).

A single RCT evaluated the effect on long-term neurodevelopmental outcomes. The quality of evidence for this outcome was graded as low. There was no significant difference in the mental development Two RCTs ascertained the effect of routine zinc supplementation on anthropometric status at 12 months of age. The quality of evidence was graded as moderate. There was no difference in the risk of underweight between the supplemented and control groups (pooled RR 1.0, 95% CI 0.92 to 1.09).

In conclusion, routine zinc supplementation does not reduce the risk of mortality, severe morbidity (diarrhoeal episodes), and malnutrition during infancy in term LBW infants. (See GRADE profile, **Table 10**.)

Balance of benefits and harms, values and preferences, and costs: There is moderate to low quality evidence for no benefits or harm in any of the critical outcomes following zinc supplementation.

Considering the costs involved in providing daily zinc supplements and the evidence for lack of benefits, policy-makers and health-care providers are unlikely to give high value to routine zinc supplementation in LBW infants.

▪ RECOMMENDATION 10

Routine zinc supplementation for LBW infants who are fed mother's own milk or donor human milk is not recommended, because there is not enough evidence of benefits to support such a recommendation.

(Weak recommendation, based on moderate to low quality evidence for lack of benefits)

Table 10. GRADE profile summary for Question 10[60-64]

(see annexes for detailed GRADE profiles and summary tables of individual studies)

OUTCOME	No. of studies	Design	Limitations in methods	Precision	Consistency	General-izability/ directness	Overall quality of evidence	Pooled effect size (95% CI) *or range of effect sizes if pooling not possible at all*
Mortality (to 1 year in one study and 6 months in another)	2	RCTs	No serious limitations	Pooled effect not significant, with wide CI	Only two studies, ES of only one consistent with no effect	Both studies from developing country settings	**LOW**	OR 0.95 (0.52, 1.74)
			(0)	(-1.0)	(-1.0)	(0)	(Total -2.0)	
Severe morbidity – diarrhoeal illness (1-week period prevalence at 12 months of age in 1, up to 6 months in 1, up to 12 months in 1)	3	RCTs	No serious limitations	Pooled effect not significant, with wide CI	Pooled ES indicates no effect, but ES of only one study consistent with no effect	All studies from developing country settings	**LOW**	RR 0.94 (0.82, 1.07)
			(0)	(-1.0)	(-1.0)	(0)	(Total -2.0)	
Neuro-development (mental development score at 12 months)	1	RCT	Limitations in follow-up	Effect not significant, with wide CI	Single study	Study from developing country setting	**LOW**	MD -2.4 points (-7.2, 2.4)
			(-0.5)	(-1.0)	(-1.0)	(0)	(Total -2.5)	
Anthropometric status - underweight or any grade of malnutrition (at 12 months)	2	RCTs	No serious limitations	Pooled effect not significant, and both CI limits exclude meaningful benefit or unacceptable harm	Only two studies, ES of only one consistent with no effect	Both studies from developing country settings	**MODERATE**	RR 1.0 (0.92, 1.09)
			(0)	(0)	(-1.0)	(0)	(Total -1.0)	

QUESTION 11: In LBW infants who are able to breastfeed (P), what is the effect of ***initiation of breastfeeding in the first day of life*** (I) compared with delaying breastfeeding for over 24 hours (C) on mortality, severe morbidity, neurodevelopment and anthropometric status (O)?

Summary of evidence: Two observational studies examined the effect of early initiation of breastfeeding on mortality during the neonatal period. Both of these community-based studies were conducted in developing country settings. The quality of evidence for this outcome was graded as low. The pooled effect was 42% reduction in mortality (95% CI 21% to 57%) with initiation of breastfeeding in the first day of life. There was evidence of a dose response, i.e. earlier initiation was associated with a greater benefit.

No studies were identified that evaluated the effect on any of the other critical outcomes in LBW infants.

To conclude, there is low quality evidence that initiation of breastfeeding in the first day of life is associated with a significant reduction in the risk of neonatal mortality when compared with delaying breastfeeding for more than 24 hours after birth. (See GRADE profile, **Table 11.**)

Balance of benefits and harms, values and preferences, and costs: There is evidence for significant benefit in neonatal mortality with early initiation of breastfeeding. Policy-makers, health-care providers and parents in both low- and middle-income and developed country settings are likely to give a high value to the benefits observed in neonatal mortality. The observed benefits clearly outweigh the low costs involved in implementation of early initiation of breastfeeding. Further, this recommendation would be consistent with the recommendation for the general population of neonates to initiate breastfeeding as soon as possible within the first hour after birth.

- ### RECOMMENDATION 11

LBW infants who are able to breastfeed should be put to the breast as soon as possible after birth when they are clinically stable.

(Strong recommendation, based on low quality evidence for benefits)

Table 11. GRADE profile summary for Question 11[2-3]

(see annexes for detailed GRADE profiles and summary tables of individual studies)

OUTCOME	No. of studies	Design	Limitations in methods	Precision	Consistency	General-izability/ directness	Overall quality of evidence	Pooled effect size (95% CI) *or range of effect sizes if pooling not possible at all*
Mortality (from 2 days to 28 days of age)	2	Observa-tion-al (-1)	Limitations in analysis (-0.5)	Pooled effect significant, and upper limit of CI meaningful (0)	Only two studies, and ES of both in same direction as pooled effect (-0.5)	Both from developing country settings (0)	**LOW** (Total -2.0)	OR 0.58 (0.43, 0.79)

QUESTION 12: In VLBW infants born in settings where total parenteral nutrition (TPN) is not possible (P), what is the effect of ***starting small amounts of oral feeds*** (about 10 ml/kg per day) in the first few days of life (I) compared with no enteral feeding (C) on mortality, severe morbidity, neurodevelopment and anthropometric status (O)?

Summary of evidence: Four RCTs, all from developed country settings, examined the effect of giving small feed volumes in the first week of life (trophic feeding) on mortality in VLBW infants. The quality of evidence was graded as low. No significant effect on the risk of mortality was observed (pooled RR 0.76, 95% CI 0.45 to 1.28).

Eight RCTs evaluated the effect on the risk of NEC. The quality of evidence for this outcome was graded as very low. There was no significant effect on the incidence of NEC (pooled RR 1.10, 95% CI 0.70 to 1.79).

Five RCTs examined the effect on the rate of weight gain during hospital stay. The outcome in these studies was the mean days to regain birth weight. The quality of evidence was graded as low. There was no significant difference in the outcome between the group of infants who received small volumes of feeds and the group that did not receive any feeds in the first few days of life (pooled MD -0.01 days, 95% CI -0.96 to 0.95).

Three RCTs evaluated the effect of trophic feeding on the length of hospital stay in VLBW infants. The quality of evidence for this outcome was graded as very low. There was no significant difference in the mean duration of hospital stay following trophic feeding (pooled MD -3.8 days, 95% CI -12.2 to 4.5).

Six RCTs studied the effect of minimal enteral nutrition on time to reach full enteral feeding. No significant difference in the mean number of days was observed (pooled MD -1.05 days, 95% CI -2.61 to

In conclusion, there is low to very low quality evidence that initiating small volumes of oral feeds in the first few days of life along with parenteral nutrition does not reduce or increase the risk of mortality and NEC in VLBW infants. It is also not associated with any benefits in short-term weight gain or length of hospital stay (see GRADE profile, **Table 12**).

Balance of benefits and harms, values and preferences, and costs: There is evidence for no significant benefits or harms in any of the critical and non-critical outcomes with feeding small volumes of human milk orally in the first week of life in VLBW infants.

Enteral fasting for even a few days has been shown to induce mucosal atrophy, decrease the secretion of gut hormones and enzymes, and impair mucosal immunity in both animals and human infants. Moreover, keeping the infants *nil per oral* in the first week of life means that they have to be given TPN. Most health facilities in low- and middle-income country settings would not have the necessary infrastructure to administer TPN. If these infants can be started on small volumes of oral feeds (along with intravenous fluids), one can possibly avoid using TPN in such settings. Also, the costs involved in implementing this intervention are not likely to be different from giving infants only intravenous fluids.

Given these considerations and the evidence for no significant harms, policy-makers and health-care providers from low- and middle-income country settings are likely to give high value to initiation of oral feeds in small amounts (trophic feeding) in the first few days of life in VLBW infants. In view of the advantages of breast milk (Recommendations 1 and 2) these small feeds should be breast milk wherever possible.

- **RECOMMENDATION 12**

VLBW infants should be given 10ml/kg per day of enteral feeds, preferably expressed breast milk, starting from the first day of life, with the remaining fluid requirement met by intravenous fluids.

(Weak situational recommendation relevant to resource-limited settings where TPN is not possible, based on low to very low quality evidence for no harm in critical outcomes)

Table 12. GRADE profile summary for Question 12[65-73]

(see annexes for detailed GRADE profiles and summary tables of individual studies)

OUTCOME	No. of studies	Design	Limitations in methods	Precision	Consistency	General-izability/ directness	Overall quality of evidence	Pooled effect size (95% CI) or range of effect sizes if pooling not possible at all
Mortality (until discharge)	4	RCTs (0)	No serious limitations (0)	Pooled effect not significant, with wide CI (-1.0)	ES of studies with <75% of total weight in the same direction as pooled effect (-1.0)	All studies from developed country settings (-0.5)	**LOW** (Total -2.5)	RR 0.76 (0.45, 1.28)
Severe morbidity – NEC (until discharge)	8	RCTs (0)	Limitations in analysis (-0.5)	Pooled effect not significant, with wide CI (-1.0)	Pooled ES indicates no effect, but ES of none of the individual studies consistent with no effect (-1.0)	Majority of evidence from studies in developed country settings (-0.5)	**VERY LOW** (Total -3.0)	RR 1.10 (0.70, 1.79)
Days to regain birth weight (during initial hospital stay)	5	RCTs (0)	Limitations in allocation of subjects and analysis (-1.0)	Pooled effect not significant, but both CI limits exclude meaningful benefit or unacceptable harm (0)	Pooled ES indicates no effect, but ES of studies with <75% of the total weight consistent with no effect (-1.0)	Majority of evidence from studies in developed country settings (-0.5)	**LOW** (Total -2.5)	MD -0.01 days (-0.96, 0.95)
Length of hospital stay	3	RCTs (0)	Limitations in outcome measurement (-0.5)	Pooled effect not significant, with wide CI (-1.0)	ES of studies with <75% of the total weight in the same direction as pooled effect (-1.0)	All the studies from developed country settings (-0.5)	**VERY LOW** (Total -3.0)	MD -6.1 days (-21.0, 8.7)

QUESTION 13: In LBW infants, what is the effect of *exclusive breastfeeding for 6 months* (I) compared with an exclusive breastfeeding duration of 4 months or less (C) on mortality, severe morbidity, neurodevelopment and anthropometric status (O)?

Summary of evidence: No studies were identified that evaluated the effect of duration of exclusive breastfeeding on mortality in LBW infants.

One cluster-RCT examining the effect of community-based promotion of exclusive breastfeeding on episodes of diarrhoeal illness during infancy was identified. Exclusive breastfeeding rates at 6 months of age in the intervention and control clusters were 41% and 4% respectively. The quality of evidence for this outcome was graded as low. There was no significant effect on the proportion of infants with diarrhoeal episodes between 3 and 6 months of age (OR 0.73, 95% CI 0.41 to 1.40). Another study, a quasi-RCT from a developing country setting, found a significant reduction in the percentage of days ill with diarrhoea between 4 and 6 months of age in term LBW infants (mean [SD]: 5.4 [8.5] days and 2.8 [5.4] days in infants who were exclusively breastfed for 6 and 4 months of age respectively; P<0.05).

Three RCTs examined the effect of exclusive breastfeeding duration of 6 months on significant anaemia at 6 months of age. The quality of evidence for this outcome was graded as very low. No significant effect on the incidence of anaemia was observed in infants who were exclusively breastfed until 6 months of age (pooled OR 1.38, 95% CI 0.81 to 2.35). Two of the three included studies supplemented infants with iron in addition to breast milk, but the largest study did not use any iron supplements.

One observational study ascertained the effect of breastfeeding duration on IQ scores at 7-8 years of age. The quality of evidence was graded as very low. The study found no significant difference in mean verbal IQ scores between infants who were exclusively breastfed for 4 to 7 months and those who were breastfed for less than 4 months (MD 2.0 points, 95% CI -4.4 to 8.4). Another study, a quasi-RCT, found no difference in either the proportion of infants walking by 12 months of age (RR 0.68, 95% CI 0.32 to 1.44) or the mean age at crawling between the two groups (MD -0.6 months, 95% CI -1.3 to 0.1).

The cluster-RCT on community-based promotion of exclusive breastfeeding that evaluated the effect on diarrhoeal illness also assessed the effect of the intervention on anthropometric status at 6 months of age. The quality of evidence was graded as very low. There was no difference in the proportions of infants with stunting (difference in proportion 9%, 95% CI -2 to 20%) or wasting (difference in proportion -2%, 95% CI -6% to 1%) at 6 months of age.

In conclusion, there is very low quality evidence that exclusive breastfeeding for 6 months compared with 4 months does not have a beneficial or harmful effect on anaemia at 6 months or mental development scores at 7-8 years of age. There is low quality evidence from a single study of breastfeeding promotion that there is no benefit or harm in terms of diarrhoeal morbidity or malnutrition. However, in this study an exclusive breastfeeding rate of only 41% was achieved at 6 months in the 'intervention' group. (See GRADE profile, **Table 13**.)

Balance of benefits and harms, values and preferences, and costs: There is low to very low quality evidence for no benefits or harms in long-term neurodevelopment, anthropometric status, significant anaemia or diarrhoeal morbidity.

The costs involved in starting complementary feeding from 4 months of age are higher than continuing exclusive breastfeeding until 6 months age. The risk of contamination involved in preparation of complementary foods is also a major consideration in low- and middle-income country settings. Further, the current global policy recommendation is to exclusively breastfeed all infants for 6 months. The available evidence does not justify a different recommendation for LBW infants. Given these

RECOMMENDATION 13

LBW infants should be exclusively breastfed until 6 months of age.

(Strong recommendation based on very low quality evidence for no harm in critical outcomes and the lower costs involved)

Table 13. GRADE profile summary for Question 13[18, 74-78]

(see annexes for detailed GRADE profiles and summary tables of individual studies)

OUTCOME	No. of studies	Design	Limitations in methods	Precision	Consistency	General-izability/ directness	Overall quality of evidence	Pooled effect size (95% CI) or range of effect sizes if pooling not possible at all
Proportion of infants with diarrhoeal episodes (between 3 and 6 months of age)	1	Cluster-RCT (0)	No serious limitations (0)	Effect not significant, with wide CI (-1.0)	Single study (-1.0)	From developing country setting (0)	**LOW** (Total -2.0)	Adjusted OR 0.73 (0.41, 1.40)
Severe morbidity – Significant anaemia (at 6 months of age)	3	Majority of evidence from observa-tional study (-1.0)	Limitations in follow-up and analysis (-1.0)	Pooled effect not significant, with wide CI (-1.0)	Effect size of two studies with ≥75% of the total weight in the same direction as the pooled effect (0)	All studies from developing country settings (0)	**VERY LOW** (Total -3.0)	Pooled OR 1.38 (0.81, 2.35)
Neurodevelopment (verbal IQ score at 7-8 years of age)	1	Observa-tional (-1.0)	Limitations in measurement (-0.5)	Effect not significant, with wide CI (-1.0)	Single study (-1.0)	From developed country setting (0)	**VERY LOW** (Total -3.5)	Adjusted MD 2.0 points (-4.4, 8.4)
Anthropometric status (at 6 months of age)	1	RCT (0)	No serious limitations (0)	Effect not significant, with wide CI (-1.0)	Single study (-1.0)	From developing country setting (0)	**LOW** (Total -2.0)	Adjusted difference in proportions for stunting: 9% (-2%, 20%) wasting: -2% (-6%, 1%)

QUESTION 14: In LBW infants who need to be fed by an alternative oral feeding method (P), what is the effect of *feeding by cup* (I) compared with bottle-feeding (C) on mortality, severe morbidity, neurodevelopment and anthropometric status (O)?

Summary of evidence: No studies were identified that compared the effects of different alternative oral feeding methods on mortality, severe morbidity such as infections, neurodevelopment, or long-term anthropometric status in LBW infants.

Three RCTs studied the effects of cup- versus bottle-feeding on the rates of exclusive breastfeeding at hospital discharge. The quality of evidence for this outcome was graded as moderate. The breastfeeding rates were significantly higher in infants fed by cup than in those fed by bottle (pooled OR 1.80, 95% CI 1.12 to 2.91). Two RCTs evaluated the effects of cup- and bottle-feeding on any breastfeeding (exclusive or partial) at 3 months after hospital discharge. The quality of evidence for this outcome was low. There was no significant difference between the two groups (pooled OR 1.43, 95% CI 0.87 to 2.34).

One RCT from a developing country setting studied the effects of cup- and bottle-feeding on short-term weight gain. The quality of evidence for this outcome was graded as low. There was no significant difference in the rate of weight gain in the 1-week period after enrolment between the two groups of infants (MD 0.6 g/kg per day, 95% CI -3.2 to 2.0).

One RCT from a developed country compared the effects of cup- and bottle-feeding on length of hospital stay in LBW infants. The quality of evidence for this outcome was graded as low. Infants in the cup-feeding group had a significantly longer hospital stay than those in the bottle-feeding group (MD 10.1 days, 95% CI 3.9 to 16.3).

One RCT examined the effects of cup- and bottle-feeding on the proportion of infants with desaturation and/or apnoea during feeding. The quality of evidence for this outcome was graded as low. The proportion was significantly less in the cup-feeding group (OR 0.29, 95% CI 0.08 to 0.99). Another study, a cross-over study from a developed country setting, also found a significant reduction in the proportion of episodes of desaturation with cup- feeding (mean [SD]: 0.05 [0.09] versus 0.13 [0.22] in cup- and bottle-feeding groups respectively; P=0.02).

There is some evidence for less spilling and greater consumption when a *palladai* is used compared with a regular cup.

In conclusion, there is moderate to low quality evidence that cup-feeding improves exclusive breastfeeding rates at discharge and reduces the risk of apnoeic episodes during feeding. On the other hand, it was associated with prolonged hospital stay, and the benefit in breastfeeding rates was not sustained at 3 months of age. (See GRADE profile, **Table 14**).

Balance of benefits and harms, values and preferences, and costs: There is no evidence for benefits in any of the critical outcomes but some evidence for benefits in non-critical outcomes, such as exclusive breastfeeding rates, with cup-feeding. There is low quality evidence for harm in another non-critical outcome (length of hospital stay).

Since cups are much easier to clean than bottles, feeding by a cup could potentially reduce the risk of severe infections, such as diarrhoea, a major consideration in low- and middle-income countries. Given that cup-feeding is also associated with benefits in breastfeeding rates, policy-makers and health-care providers from resource-limited settings are likely to give a high value to this feeding method. On the other hand, the possible effect on duration of hospital stay might increase the costs and effort involved

RECOMMENDATION 14

LBW infants who need to be fed by an alternative oral feeding method should be fed by cup (or *palladai* which is a cup with a beak) or spoon.

(Strong situational recommendation relevant to resource-limited settings, based on moderate quality evidence for benefits in a non-critical outcome)

Table 14. GRADE profile summary for Question 14[79-84]

(see annexes for detailed GRADE profiles and summary tables of individual studies)

OUTCOME	No. of studies	Design	Limitations in methods	Precision	Consistency	Generaliz-ability/ directness	Overall quality of evidence	Pooled effect size (95% CI) *or range of effect sizes if pooling not possible at all*
Exclusive breastfeed-ing (at discharge)	3	RCTs (0)	Limitations in measurement (-0.5)	Pooled effect significant and lower limit of CI meaningful (0)	ES of two studies with ≥75% of total weight in same direction as pooled effect (0)	All studies from developed country settings (-0.5)	**MODERATE** (Total -1.0)	OR 1.80 (1.12, 2.91)
Any breastfeed-ing (at 3 months after discharge)	2	RCTs (0)	Limitations in measurement (-0.5)	Pooled effect not significant, with wide CI (-1.0)	Only two studies, ES of both in same direction (-0.5)	Most evidence from developed country setting (-0.5)	**LOW** (Total -2.5)	OR 1.43 (0.87, 2.34)
Weight gain (during the 1 week period after enrolment)	1	RCT (0)	Limitations in analysis (-0.5)	Effect not significant, with wide CI (-1.0)	Single study (-1.0)	From developing country setting (0)	**LOW** (Total -2.5)	MD -0.6 g/kg/day (-3.2, 2.0)
Length of hospital stay	1	RCT (0)	Limitations in measurement (-0.5)	Effect significant, lower limit of CI also meaningful (0)	Single study (-1.0)	From developed country setting (-0.5)	**LOW** (Total -2.0)	MD 10.1 days (3.9, 16.3)
Apnoeic episodes (during feeding)	1	RCT (0)	Limitations in analysis (-0.5)	Effect significant, but upper limit of CI close to null (-0.5)	Single study (-1.0)	From developing country setting (0)	**LOW** (Total -2.0)	OR 0.29 (0.08, 0.99)

QUESTION 15: In VLBW infants who need to be given intragastric tube feeding (P), what is the effect of ***bolus intermittent feeding*** (I) compared with continuous feeding (C) on mortality, severe morbidity, neurodevelopment and anthropometric status (O)?

Summary of evidence: No studies were found that compared the effects of intermittent feeding and continuous feeding through intragastric tube on mortality in VLBW infants.

Four studies (three RCTs and one quasi-RCT, all from developed country settings) compared the effects of bolus and continuous intragastric tube feeding on NEC. The quality of evidence for this outcome was graded as low. There was no significant difference in the incidence of NEC between the two feeding groups (RR 0.99, 95% CI 0.51 to 1.92). However, the CI is wide, and therefore the result should be interpreted with caution.

A total of four RCTs evaluated the effect on rate of weight gain during hospital stay. The outcome assessed was the number of days to regain birth weight. The quality of evidence was graded as very low. No significant difference was found between the groups of infants receiving bolus feeding and continuous intragastric tube feeding (MD -0.46 days, 95% CI -1.48 to 0.55).

Five RCTs ascertained the effects of bolus and continuous intragastric tube feeding on the number of days to reach full feeds. The quality of evidence for this outcome was graded as low. There was no significant difference between the two groups (MD -1.86 days, 95% CI -5.8 to 2.1).

One RCT studied the effects on the number of apnoeic episodes during feeding. The quality of evidence was graded as low. There was no significant difference between the two feeding groups in the number of episodes during the entire study period (MD -14.0 episodes, 95% CI -28.2 to 0.2). Another study, an RCT from a developed country setting, also found no significant difference in the number of apnoeic episodes per day between the two groups (MD 0.6 episodes, 95% CI -0.79 to 1.99).

In conclusion, there is low to very low quality evidence that bolus or intermittent feeding and continuous feeding through intragastric tube are not different in the risk of NEC, days to regain birth weight or days to reach full feeds when compared with continuous feeding. (See GRADE profile, **Table 15.**)

Balance of benefits and harms, values and preferences, and costs: There is evidence for no significant benefits or harms in any of the critical and non-critical outcomes with bolus intragastric tube feeding.

Unlike continuous intragastric tube feeding, bolus or intermittent feeding does not require syringe pumps or other infusion pumps. Implementing bolus feeding might therefore be associated with lower costs than implementing continuous feeding. Given that there is no difference in benefits or harm between the two methods, policy-makers and health-care providers are likely to give high value to bolus, intermittent feeding through intragastric tube in VLBW infants.

- ### RECOMMENDATION 15

VLBW infants requiring intragastric tube feeding should be given bolus intermittent feeds.

(Weak recommendation, based on low to very low quality evidence for no difference in benefits or harm but lower costs)

Table 15. GRADE profile summary for Question 15[67, 85-89]

(see annexes for detailed GRADE profiles and summary tables of individual studies)

OUTCOME	No. of studies	Design	Limitations in methods	Precision	Consistency	Generaliza bility/ directness	Overall quality of evidence	Pooled effect size (95% CI) or range of effect sizes if pooling not possible at all
Severe morbidity – NEC (during initial hospital stay)	4 (3 RCTs; 1 quasi-RCT)	Majority of evidence from RCTs (0)	No serious limitations (0)	Pooled effect not significant, with wide CI (-1.0)	Pooled ES indicates no effect but ES of only one study is consistent with no effect (-1.0)	All studies from developed country settings (-0.5)	**LOW** (Total -2.5)	RR 0.99 (0.51, 1.92)
Days to regain birth weight (during initial hospital stay)	4	RCTs (0)	Limitations in analysis (-0.5)	Pooled effect not significant, with wide CI (-1.0)	Pooled ES indicates no effect, and ES of studies with <75% of total weight is consistent with no effect (-1.0)	All studies from developed country settings (-0.5)	**VERY LOW** (Total -3.0)	MD -0.46 days (-1.48, 0.55)
Days to reach full feeds (during initial hospital stay)	5	RCTs (0)	Limitations in measurement and analysis (-1.0)	Pooled effect not significant, with wide CI (-1.0)	ES of 4 studies with ≥75% of total weight in the same direction as the pooled ES (0)	All studies from developed country settings (-0.5)	**LOW** (Total -2.5)	MD -1.86 days (-5.8, 2.1)
Apnoeic episodes during feeding (during initial hospital stay)	1	RCT (0)	No serious limitations (0)	Effect not significant, with wide CI (-1.0)	Single study (-1.0)	From developed country setting (-0.5)	**LOW** (Total -2.5)	MD -14.0 episodes (-28.2, 0.2)

QUESTION 16: In VLBW infants who need to be given intragastric tube feeding (P), what is the effect of *orogastric tube feeding* (I) compared with nasogastric tube feeding (C) on mortality, severe morbidity, neurodevelopment and anthropometric status (O)?

Summary of evidence: No studies were found that examined the effects of the different routes of intragastric tube placement (oral and nasal) on mortality, neurodevelopment and long-term growth in VLBW infants. Indeed, only one RCT was identified that ascertained the effects of oral and nasal routes of tube placement on severe morbidities and growth during hospital stay. This study found no significant differences in either the risk of NEC (RR 2.78, 95% CI 0.12 to 50.0), mean number of days to regain birth weight (MD -0.9 days, 95% CI -3.1 to 1.3) or in the duration of oxygen supplementation (MD -7.6 days, 95% CI -30.4 to 15.2) between the orogastric and nasogastric tube feeding groups. The quality of evidence for all three outcomes was graded as very low.

A descriptive study from a developed country setting reported a significant increase in nasal resistance and total airway resistance following insertion of a nasogastric tube in preterm infants born before 32 weeks gestation. There were, however, no differences in either the nasal resistance or total airway resistance between the nasogastric and orogastric tube feeding groups at one month after removal of the tubes.

In conclusion, there is very low quality evidence that orogastric tube feeding does not reduce the risk of NEC, days to regain birth weight or the duration of oxygen supplementation when compared with nasogastric tube feeding. (See GRADE profile, **Table 16**).

Balance of benefits and harms, values and preferences, and costs: There is no evidence for benefits or harms in any of the critical outcomes with orogastric tube feeding compared with nasogastric tube feeding.

Orogastric tubes are easier to insert but are relatively more difficult to fix than tubes placed through the nasal route. This might result in frequent change of feeding tubes, thereby increasing the costs. On the other hand, nasogastric tube feeding has been associated with some deterioration in physiological parameters, such as airway resistance, and carries a risk of injury to the nasal mucosa. Therefore, policy-makers, health-care providers, and parents are likely to be equivocal regarding the optimal route of placement of an intragastric tube.

▪ RECOMMENDATION 16

In VLBW infants who need to be given intragastric tube feeding, the intragastric tube may be placed either by the oral or nasal route, depending upon the preferences of health-care providers.

(Weak recommendation, based on lack of evidence for benefits or harm in any of the critical outcomes)

Table 16. GRADE profile summary for Question 16[86, 90]

(see annexes for detailed GRADE profiles and summary tables of individual studies)

OUTCOME	No. of studies	Design	Limitations in methods	Precision	Consistency	General-izability/ directness	Overall quality of evidence	Pooled effect size (95% CI) or range of effect sizes if pooling not possible at all
Severe morbidity – NEC	1	RCT (0)	Limitations in analysis (-0.5)	Pooled effect not significant, with wide CI (-1.0)	Single study (-1.0)	From developed country setting (-0.5)	**VERY LOW** (Total -3.0)	RR 2.78 (0.12, 50.0)
Days to regain birth weight (during initial hospital stay)	1	RCT (0)	Limitations in measurement and analysis (-1.0)	Pooled effect not significant, with wide CI (-1.0)	Single study (-1.0)	From developed country setting (-0.5)	**VERY LOW** (Total -3.5)	MD -0.9 days (-3.1, 1.3)
Duration of oxygen supplement ation (during initial hospital stay)	1	RCT (0)	Limitations in measurement and analysis (-1.0)	Pooled effect not significant, with wide CI (-1.0)	Single study (-1.0)	From developed country setting (-0.5)	**VERY LOW** (Total -3.5)	MD -7.6 days (-30.4, 15.2)

QUESTION 17: In LBW infants who are fully or mostly fed by an alternative oral feeding method (P), what is the effect of *feeding based on infants' hunger cues* (I) compared with strict scheduled feeding (C) on mortality, severe morbidity, neurodevelopment and anthropometric status (O)?

Summary of evidence: No studies compared the effects of feeding based on infants' hunger cues and those of scheduled feeding on mortality, severe morbidity including hypoglycemia, neurodevelopment or anthropometric status (at or beyond 6 months of age). A Cochrane review included eight RCTs, all from developed country settings, involving 496 infants in total. One additional study was found (observational, from developed country settings). Feeding was initiated in response to infants' hunger cues in all studies and was stopped based on satiation cues or after a prescribed volume was administered. In many of these studies, infants were aroused to feed orally if they did not demonstrate Three studies (two RCTs and one observational) have ascertained the effects of feeding based on infants' hunger cues and scheduled feeding on weight gain during hospital stay. The quality of evidence for this outcome was graded as very low. There was no significant difference in the mean weight gain between the two groups (MD -0.47 g/kg per day, 95% CI -3.76 to 2.82). Another study, an RCT not included in the meta-analysis, also reported no difference in the mean weight gain between the two groups of infants (MD -2.8 g per day, 95% CI -6.55, 0.95). The other five studies also examined the effect on short-term growth. However, they could not be included in the meta-analysis because of incomplete data. Four of these studies reported no significant differences in the rate of weight gain during the study period; the fifth study reported the mean daily weight gain in both the groups (26.4 g versus 34.1 g) but did not elaborate as to whether the difference was statistically significant.

Three RCTs evaluated the effect of feeding based on hunger cues on the length of hospital stay. The quality of evidence for this outcome was graded as moderate. The pooled MD in the postmenstrual age at discharge was 0.55 weeks shorter (95% CI -0.84, -0.26) in those receiving feeding based on hunger cues. However, these results have to be interpreted with caution, because the largest study included in the meta-analysis used a co-intervention (non-nutritive sucking) known to shorten the length of hospital stay in preterm infants. As with the previous outcome, the data from five RCTs were not included in the meta-analysis because of incomplete data. Of these, three studies reported no significant difference in either the mean duration of hospital stay or mean age at discharge while one study reported a significant difference in the number of days from enrolment until infants were ready for discharge (2.7 versus 8.9 days; P value not reported). The fifth study reported the duration of hospital stay in the two groups (31 versus 33 days) but did not mention whether the difference was statistically significant.

Two RCTs studied the effect of feeding based on infants' hunger cues on time to reach full feeds in preterm infants. The quality of evidence for this outcome was graded as moderate. The pooled MD is 2.8 days less (95% CI -3.6, -2.1) in infants who received feeding based on hunger cues. Another RCT reported that infants in the group fed based on hunger cues achieved full feeds earlier than the control group infants (2.7 versus 8.9 days), but did not comment on the statistical significance.

In conclusion, there is moderate quality evidence that feeding based on infants' hunger cues reduces the time to reach full enteral feeds and possibly the length of hospital stay. There is very low quality evidence that it does not increase the rate of weight gain during initial hospital stay. (See GRADE profile, **Table 17**).

Balance of benefits and harms, values and preferences, and costs: There is no evidence of benefits or harms in any of the critical outcomes. Policy-makers, health-care providers and parents are likely to value shorter hospital stays, but this observed benefit could have been confounded by another intervention (non-nutritive sucking). Since feeding based on infants' hunger cues requires a greater number of well-trained health providers to feed the babies and train the mothers to look for hunger cues, implementing this approach would be associated with higher costs.

- **RECOMMENDATION 17**

LBW infants who are fully or mostly fed by an alternative oral feeding method should be fed based on infants' hunger cues, except when the infant remains asleep beyond 3 hours since the last feed.

(Weak situational recommendation relevant to settings with adequate number of health care providers, based on moderate to low quality evidence for benefit in non-critical outcomes)

Table 17. GRADE profile summary for Question 17[91-100]

(see annexes for detailed GRADE tables and summary tables of individual studies)

OUTCOME	No. of studies	Design	Limitations in methods	Precision	Consistency	General-izability/ directness	Overall quality of evidence	Pooled effect size (95% CI) or range of effect sizes if pooling not possible at all
Weight gain (during initial hospital stay)	3 (2 RCTs, 1 observa-tional) (0)	Majority of evidence from RCTs	Limitations in allocation of subjects (-0.5)	Pooled effect not significant, with wide CI (-1.0)	Pooled ES indicates no effect but ES of only one study is consistent with no effect (-1.0)	All studies from developed country settings (-0.5)	**VERY LOW** (Total -3.0)	MD -0.47 g/kg/day (-3.76, 2.82)
Age at discharge (post-menstrual or post-conceptional age)	3	RCTs (0)	Limitations in measurement (-0.5)	Pooled effect significant, upper limit also meaningful (0)	ES of studies with ≥75% of total weight in same direction as pooled ES (0)	All studies from developed country settings (-0.5)	**MODERATE** (Total -1.0)	MD -0.55 weeks (-0.84, -0.26)
Days to reach full oral feeds (after trial entry)	2	RCTs (0)	Limitations in measurement (-0.5)	Pooled effect significant and upper limit of CI meaningful (0)	Only two studies, both in the same direction (-0.5)	Both from developed country settings (-0.5)	**MODERATE** (Total -1.5)	MD -2.8 days (-3.6, -2.1)

QUESTION 18: In VLBW infants who need to be fed by an alternative oral feeding method or given intragastric feeds (P), what is the effect of rapid (≥30 ml/kg per day) progression of feeds (I) compared with slow (≤20 ml/kg per day) progression (C) on mortality, severe morbidity, neurodevelopment and anthropometric status (O)?

Summary of evidence: Three RCTs evaluated the effect of rapid progression of feeds (≥30 ml/kg per day) on mortality in VLBW infants. Two of the studies were from developing country settings. The quality of evidence for this outcome was graded as moderate. There was no significant difference in the risk of mortality between the 'fast' and 'slow' feeding groups (pooled RR 0.67, 95% CI 0.36 to 1.22).

Four RCTs – two each from developed and developing country settings – examined the effect of rapid progression of enteral feeds on the incidence of NEC. The quality of evidence for this outcome was graded as low. There was no significant difference in the risk of NEC between the two groups, but the wide CI means that this finding is inconclusive (pooled RR 1.02, 95% CI 0.51 to 2.05).

No studies were found that examined the effects of rapid and slow progression of feeds on neurodevelopment and anthropometric status at 6 months of age or more in preterm LBW infants. We included four RCTs that studied the effects of rapid and slow progression of feeds on weight gain during initial hospital stay. Since the studies reported only median and range/inter-quartile ranges, the results could not be pooled. The quality of evidence for this outcome was graded as high. All four studies showed a significant reduction in the median days to regain birth weight – the reported median difference ranging from 2 to 6 days.

Three RCTs have looked at the effect of rapid feed progression on the duration of hospital stay in LBW infants. The results of these studies were also not pooled (only median and ranges available). The quality of evidence for this outcome was graded as low. Infants in the rapid feeding group from all the studies had shorter duration of stay in the hospital; however, the difference was not statistically significant in two studies. The third study reported a significant difference between the two groups (median [range] 9.5 days [8.4 to 13.8] versus 11.0 [10.0 to 15.0]; P<0.005).

In conclusion, there is moderate to low quality evidence that rapid progression of oral feeds does not reduce or increase the risk of mortality or NEC. The only benefit is that it reduces the time to regain birth weight in VLBW infants. (See GRADE profile, **Table 18**).

Balance of benefits and harms, values and preferences, and costs: There is no evidence of benefits or harms in any of the critical outcomes, but some benefit was observed in one 'other' non-critical outcome (rate of weight gain during hospital stay).

The benefit in short-term weight gain is likely to be given some value by parents and health-care providers. However, policy-makers are unlikely to give a high value to this benefit in the absence of evidence of benefit on critical outcomes. The costs of implementing faster progression of feeding are

RECOMMENDATION 18

In VLBW infants who need to be fed by an alternative oral feeding method or given intragastric tube feeds, feed volumes can be increased by up to 30 ml/kg per day with careful monitoring for feed intolerance.

(Weak recommendation, based on high quality evidence for benefit in a non-critical outcome)

Table 18. GRADE profile summary for Question 18[101-104]

(see annexes for detailed GRADE profiles and summary tables of individual studies)

OUTCOME	No. of studies	Design	Limitations in methods	Precision	Consistency	General-izability/ directness	Overall quality of evidence	Pooled effect size (95% CI) or range of effect sizes if pooling not possible at all
Mortality (until discharge)	3	RCTs	No serious limitations (0)	Pooled effect not significant, with wide CI (-1.0)	ES of two studies with ≥75% of total weight in same direction as pooled ES (0)	Majority of evidence from studies in developing country settings (0)	**MODERATE** (Total - 1.0)	RR 0.67 (0.36, 1.22)
Severe morbidity – NEC	4	RCTs	No serious limitations (0)	Pooled effect not significant, with wide CI (-1.0)	Pooled ES indicates no effect but ES of none of the individual studies is consistent with no effect (-1.0)	Majority of evidence from studies in developed country settings (-0.5)	**LOW** (Total - 2.5)	RR 1.02 (0.51, 2.05)
Days to regain birth weight (during initial hospital stay)	4	RCTs	No serious limitations (0)	4/4 studies significant (0)	ES of all studies in the same direction (0)	Majority of evidence from studies in developed country settings (-0.5)	**HIGH** (Total - 0.5)	Range of median differences: -6 to -2 days
Duration of hospital stay	3	RCTs	Limitations in measurement (-0.5)	2/3 studies not significant (-1.0)	All 3 studies in the same direction (0)	Majority of evidence from studies in developed country settings (-0.5)	**LOW** (Total - 2.0)	Range of median differences: -3 to -1.5 days

FIELD TESTING OF GUIDELINES

Recommendations for feeding LBW infants were first drafted in 2006, and a set of training materials for health workers who care for LBW infants was developed based on these recommendations. A field test with a pre-post design was conducted in two district-level hospitals each in Ghana, India, Pakistan and Uganda in 2008-9. The objectives of the field test were to evaluate the feasibility and acceptability of implementing the guidelines and to document the effect of guideline implementation on the knowledge and skills of health workers and mothers. The relatively small sample size of 120 infants per country was not sufficient to detect improvements in feeding practices.

In all countries, health providers who care for LBW infants were trained in a 3-day workshop comprised of self-reading sessions and classroom demonstrations using video and posters based on the guidelines, combined with clinical demonstrations and practice. A typical workshop included about 20 participants and 2-4 facilitators/trainers. In addition to training, supervision and on- the-job support was provided to the health workers, and efforts were made to improve facilities and supplies where possible.

The results of the field tests in all four countries were very encouraging. It was feasible to implement the guidelines in all the sites, and they were found to be acceptable to health workers and mothers. Both the health workers and mothers felt that implementation of the guidelines had improved the care of LBW infants. Finally, there was a substantial and statistically significant improvement in knowledge and skills of health providers related to optimal feeding of LBW infants in all the study sites.

IMPLEMENTATION PLAN

These guidelines will be disseminated to Ministries of Health of relevant countries through the WHO Regional and Country offices. The draft training materials related to the guidelines, including the reading materials for sessions, posters and video, will be finalized and made available to countries through WHO Regional and Country Offices as reference material. However, the main implementation strategy for these guidelines and training materials will be through incorporation into the flagship tools and training materials of the Department of Maternal, Newborn, Child and Adolescent Health, including IMCI and Integrated management of pregnancy and childbirth (IMPAC) materials for community, first-level health facilities and referral hospitals. These materials are already in use in over 100 countries.

REFERENCES

Introduction and methodology sections:

I. WHO, UNICEF. *Low birthweight: country, regional and global estimates*. Geneva, UNICEF and WHO, 2004.

II. Lawn JE et al. 4 million neonatal deaths: When? Where? Why? *Lancet*, 2005, 365(9462):891–900.

III. Ashworth A. Effects of intrauterine growth retardation on mortality and morbidity in infants and young children. *European Journal of Clinical Nutrition*, 1998, 52 Supplement 1:S34–41.

IV. McCormick MC. The contribution of low birth weight to infant mortality and childhood morbidity. *New England Journal of Medicine*, 1985, 312:82–90.

V. Fryer JG, Ashford JR. Trends in perinatal and neonatal mortality in England and Wales 1960–69. *British Journal of Preventive and Social Medicine*, 1972, 26(1):1–9.

VI. Lawn JE et al. 'Kangaroo mother care' to prevent neonatal deaths due to pre-term birth complications. *International Journal of Epidemiology*, 2010, 39:i144-154 (doi:10.1093/ije/dyq031).

VII. Bang AT et al. Low birth weight and preterm neonates: can they be managed at home by mother and a trained village health worker? *Journal of Perinatology*, 2005, 25 Supplement 1:S72-81.

VIII. Pratinidhi AK et al. Domiciliary care of low birth weight neonates. *Indian Journal of Pediatrics*, 1986, 53(1):87-92.

IX. WHO. *Pocket book of hospital care for children: guidelines for the management of common illnesses with limited resources*. Geneva, WHO, 2005.

X. WHO. *Managing newborn problems: a guide for doctors, nurses, and midwives*. Geneva, WHO, 2003.

Recommendations section:

1. Meinzen-Derr J et al. Role of human milk in extremely low birth weight infants' risk of necrotizing enterocolitis or death. *Journal of Perinatology*, 2009, 29:57-62.

2. Mullany LC et al. Breast-feeding patterns, time to initiation, and mortality risk among newborns in southern Nepal. *Journal of Nutrition*, 2008, 138:599-603.

3. Edmond KM et al. Impact of early infant feeding practices on mortality in low birth weight infants from rural Ghana. *Journal of Perinatology*, 2008, 28:438-444.

4. Chen A, Rogan WJ. Breastfeeding and the risk of postneonatal death in the United States. *Pediatrics*, 2004, 113:e435-439.

5. Narayanan I et al. Partial supplementation with expressed breast-milk for prevention of infection in low-birth-weight infants. *Lancet*, 1980,2:561-563.

6. Narayanan I, Prakash K, Gujral VV. Bacteriological analysis of expressed human milk and its relation to the outcome of high risk low birth weight infants. *Indian Pediatrics*, 1983, 20:915-920.

7. Lucas A, Cole TJ. Breast milk and neonatal necrotising enterocolitis. *Lancet,* 1990, 336:1519-1523.

8. Hylander MA, Strobino DM, Dhanireddy R. Human milk feedings and infection among very low birth weight infants. *Pediatrics*, 1998,102:E38.

9. Schanler RJ, Shulman RJ, Lau C. Feeding strategies for premature infants: beneficial outcomes of feeding fortified human milk versus preterm formula. *Pediatrics*, 1999,103:1150-1157.

10. Sisk PM et al. Early human milk feeding is associated with a lower risk of necrotizing enterocolitis in very low birth weight infants. *Journal of Perinatology*, 2007, 27:428-433.

11. Henderson G et al. Enteral feeding regimens and necrotising enterocolitis in preterm infants: a multicentre case-control study. *Archives of Disease in Childhood Fetal and Neonatal Edition*, 2009,94:F120-123.

12. Levy I et al. Urinary tract infection in preterm infants: the protective role of breastfeeding. *Pediatric Nephrology*, 2009, 24:527-531.

13. Doyle LW et al. Breastfeeding and intelligence. *Lancet,* 1992, 339:744-745.

14. Morley R et al. Mother's choice to provide breast milk and developmental outcome. *Archives of Disease in Childhood,* 1988, 63:1382-1385.

15. Morley R et al. Neurodevelopment in children born small for gestational age: a randomized trial of nutrient-enriched versus standard formula and comparison with a reference breastfed group. *Pediatrics,* 2004, 113:515-521.

16. Tanaka K et al. Does breastfeeding in the neonatal period influence the cognitive function of very-low-birth-weight infants at 5 years of age? *Brain and Development,* 2009, 31:288-293.

17. Vohr BR et al. Persistent beneficial effects of breast milk ingested in the neonatal intensive care unit on outcomes of extremely low birth weight infants at 30 months of age. *Pediatrics,* 2007, 120:e953-959.

18. Horwood LJ, Darlow BA, Mogridge N. Breast milk feeding and cognitive ability at 7-8 years. *Archives of Disease in Childhood Fetal and Neonatal Edition,* 2001, 84:F23-27.

19. Zukowsky K. Breast-fed low-birth-weight premature neonates: developmental assessment and nutritional intake in the first 6 months of life. *Journal of Perinatal and Neonatal Nursing,* 2007, 21:242-249.

20. Pollock JI. Mother's choice to provide breast milk and developmental outcome. *Archives of Disease in Childhood,* 1989, 64:763-764.

21. Lucas A et al. Randomized trial of nutrient-enriched formula versus standard formula for postdischarge preterm infants. *Pediatrics,* 2001, 108:703-711.

22. Lucas A et al. Multicentre trial on feeding low birthweight infants: effects of diet on early growth. *Archives of Disease in Childhood,* 1984, 59:722-730.

23. Schanler RJ et al. Randomized trial of donor human milk versus preterm formula as substitutes for mothers' own milk in the feeding of extremely premature infants. *Pediatrics,* 2005, 116:400-406.

24. Gross SJ. Growth and biochemical response of preterm infants fed human milk or modified infant formula. *New England Journal of Medicine,* 1983, 308:237-241.

25. Tyson JE et al. Growth, metabolic response, and development in very-low-birth-weight infants fed banked human milk or enriched formula: I. Neonatal findings. *Journal of Pediatrics,* 1983, 103:95-104.

26. Cooper PA et al. Growth and biochemical response of premature infants fed pooled preterm milk or special formula. *Journal of Pediatric Gastroenterology and Nutrition,* 1984, 3:749-754.

27. Sullivan S et al. An exclusively human milk-based diet is associated with a lower rate of necrotizing enterocolitis than a diet of human milk and bovine milk-based products. *Journal of Pediatrics,* 2010, 156:562-567.

28. Lucas A et al. Early diet of preterm infants and development of allergic or atopic disease: randomised prospective study. *British Medical Journal,* 1990, 300:837-840.

29. Lucas A, Morley R, Cole TJ. Randomised trial of early diet in preterm babies and later intelligence quotient. *British Medical Journal,* 1998, 317:1481-1487.

30. Morley R, Lucas A. Randomized diet in the neonatal period and growth performance until 7.5-8 y of age in preterm children. *American Journal of Clinical Nutrition,* 2000, 71:822-828.

31. Cooke RJ et al. Feeding preterm infants after hospital discharge: growth and development at 18 months of age. *Pediatric Research,* 2001, 49:719-722.

32. Carver JD et al. Growth of preterm infants fed nutrient-enriched or term formula after hospital discharge. *Pediatrics,* 2001, 107:683-689.

33. Koo WW, Hockman EM. Posthospital discharge feeding for preterm infants: effects of standard compared with enriched milk formula on growth, bone mass, and body composition. *American Journal of Clinical Nutrition,* 2006, 84:1357-1364.

34. Fewtrell MS et al. Catch-up growth in small-for-gestational-age term infants: a randomized trial. *American Journal of Clinical Nutrition,* 2001, 74:516-523.

35. Lucas A et al. Randomized outcome trial of human milk fortification and developmental outcome in preterm infants. *American Journal of Clinical Nutrition,* 1996, 64:142-151.

36. Pettifor JM et al. Bone mineralization and mineral homeostasis in very low-birth-weight infants fed either human milk or fortified human milk. *Journal of Pediatric Gastroenterology and Nutrition*, 1989, 8:217-224.

37. Faerk J et al. Diet and bone mineral content at term in premature infants. *Pediatric Research*, 2000, 47:148-156.

38. Kashyap S et al. Growth, nutrient retention, and metabolic response of low-birth-weight infants fed supplemented and unsupplemented preterm human milk. *American Journal of Clinical Nutrition*, 1990, 52:254-262.

39. Modanlou HD et al. Growth, biochemical status, and mineral metabolism in very-low-birth-weight infants receiving fortified preterm human milk. *Journal of Pediatric Gastroenterology and Nutrition*, 1986, 5:762-767.

40. Zuckerman M, Pettifor JM. Rickets in very-low-birth-weight infants born at Baragwanath Hospital. *South African Medical Journal*, 1994, 84:216-220.

41. Wauben IP et al. Moderate nutrient supplementation of mother's milk for preterm infants supports adequate bone mass and short-term growth: a randomized, controlled trial. *American Journal of Clinical Nutrition*, 1998, 67:465-472.

42. Greer FR, McCormick A. Improved bone mineralization and growth in premature infants fed fortified own mother's milk. *Journal of Pediatrics*, 1988, 112:961-969.

43. Carey DE et al. Growth and phosphorus metabolism in premature infants fed human milk, fortified human milk, or special premature formula. Use of serum procollagen as a marker of growth. *American Journal of Disease in Childhood*, 1987, 141:511-515.

44. Nicholl RM, Gamsu HR. Changes in growth and metabolism in very low birthweight infants fed with fortified breast milk. *Acta Paediatrica*, 1999, 88:1056-1061.

45. Polberger SK, Axelsson IA, Raiha NC. Growth of very low birth weight infants on varying amounts of human milk protein. *Pediatric Research*, 1989, 25:414-419.

46. Mukhopadhyay K, Narnag A, Mahajan R. Effect of human milk fortification in appropriate for gestation and small for gestation preterm babies: a randomized controlled trial. *Indian Pediatrics*, 2007, 44:286-290.

47. Backstrom MC et al. Randomised controlled trial of vitamin D supplementation on bone density and biochemical indices in preterm infants. *Archives of Disease in Childhood Fetal Neonatal Edition* , 1999, 80:F161-166.

48. Backstrom MC et al. The long-term effect of early mineral, vitamin D, and breast milk intake on bone mineral status in 9- to 11-year-old children born prematurely. *Journal of Pediatric Gastroenterology and Nutrition*, 1999, 29:575-582.

49. Evans JR et al. Effect of high-dose vitamin D supplementation on radiographically detectable bone disease of very low birth weight infants. *Journal of Pediatrics*, 1989, 115:779-786.

50. Holland PC et al. Prenatal deficiency of phosphate, phosphate supplementation, and rickets in very-low-birthweight infants. *Lancet*, 1990, 335:697-701.

51. McIntosh N, De Curtis M, Williams J. Failure of mineral supplementation to reduce incidence of rickets in very-low-birthweight infants. *Lancet*, 1986, 2:981-982.

52. Lucas A et al. Early diet in preterm babies and developmental status in infancy. *Archives of Disease in Childhood*, 1989, 64:1570-1578.

53. Franz AR et al. Prospective randomized trial of early versus late enteral iron supplementation in infants with a birth weight of less than 1301 grams. *Pediatrics*, 2000, 106:700-706.

54. Arnon S et al. The efficacy and safety of early supplementation of iron polymaltose complex in preterm infants. *American Journal of Perinatology*, 2007, 24:95-100.

55. Sankar MJ et al. Early iron supplementation in very low birth weight infants--a randomized controlled trial. *Acta Paediatrica*, 2009, 98:953-958.

56. Lundstrom U, Siimes MA, Dallman PR. At what age does iron supplementation become necessary in low-birth-weight infants? *Journal of Pediatrics*, 1977, 91:878-883.

57. Steinmacher J et al. Randomized trial of early versus late enteral iron supplementation in infants with a birth weight of less than 1301 grams: neurocognitive development at 5.3 years' corrected age. *Pediatrics*, 2007, 120:538-546.

58. Darlow BA, Graham PJ. Vitamin A supplementation to prevent mortality and short- and long-term morbidity in very low birthweight infants. *Cochrane Database Systematic Reviews*, 2007, CD000501.

59. Wardle SP et al. Randomised controlled trial of oral vitamin A supplementation in preterm infants to prevent chronic lung disease. *Archives of Disease in Childhood Fetal and Neonatal Edition*, 2001, 84:F9-F13.

60. Taneja S et al. Effect of zinc supplementation on morbidity and growth in hospital-born, low-birth-weight infants. *American Journal of Clinical Nutrition*, 2009, 90:385-391.

61. Lira PI, Ashworth A, Morris SS. Effect of zinc supplementation on the morbidity, immune function, and growth of low-birth-weight, full-term infants in northeast Brazil. *American Journal of Clinical Nutrition*, 1998, 68:418S-424S.

62. Sazawal S et al. Zinc supplementation in infants born small for gestational age reduces mortality: a prospective, randomized, controlled trial. *Pediatrics*, 2001,108:1280-1286.

63. Sur D et al. Impact of zinc supplementation on diarrheal morbidity and growth pattern of low birth weight infants in Kolkata, India: a randomized, double-blind, placebo-controlled, community-based study. *Pediatrics*, 2003, 112:1327-1332.

64. Ashworth A et al. Zinc supplementation, mental development and behaviour in low birth weight term infants in northeast Brazil. *European Journal of Clinical Nutrition*, 1998, 52:223-227.

65. McClure RJ, Newell SJ. Randomised controlled study of clinical outcome following trophic feeding. *Archives of Disease in Childhood Fetal and Neonatal Edition*, 2000, 82:F29-33.

66. Mosqueda E et al. The early use of minimal enteral nutrition in extremely low birth weight newborns. *Journal of Perinatology*, 2008, 28:264-269.

67. Schanler RJ et al. Feeding strategies for premature infants: randomized trial of gastrointestinal priming and tube-feeding method. *Pediatrics*, 1999, 103:434-439.

68. van Elburg RM et al. Minimal enteral feeding, fetal blood flow pulsatility, and postnatal intestinal permeability in preterm infants with intrauterine growth retardation. *Archives of Disease in Childhood Fetal Neonatal and Edition*, 2004, 89:F293-296.

69. Saenz de Pipaon M et al. Effect of minimal enteral feeding on splanchnic uptake of leucine in the postabsorptive state in preterm infants. *Pediatric Research*, 2003, 53:281-287.

70. Dunn L et al. Beneficial effects of early hypocaloric enteral feeding on neonatal gastrointestinal function: preliminary report of a randomized trial. *Journal of Pediatrics*, 1988, 112:622-629.

71. Becerra M et al. Feeding Vlbw infants: effect of early enteral stimulation (Ees). *Pediatric Research*, 1996, 39:304.

72. Troche B et al. Early minimal feedings promote growth in critically ill premature infants. *Biology of the Neonate*, 1995, 67:172-181.

73. Meetze WH et al. Gastrointestinal priming prior to full enteral nutrition in very low birth weight infants. *Journal of Pediatric Gastroenterology and Nutrition*, 1992, 15:163-170.

74. Bhandari N et al. Effect of community-based promotion of exclusive breastfeeding on diarrhoeal illness and growth: a cluster randomised controlled trial. *Lancet*, 2003, 361:1418-1423.

75. Dewey KG et al. Age of introduction of complementary foods and growth of term, low-birth-weight, breast-fed infants: a randomized intervention study in Honduras. *American Journal of Clinical Nutrition*, 1999, 69:679-686.

76. Dewey KG, Cohen RJ, Brown KH. Exclusive breast-feeding for 6 months, with iron supplementation, maintains adequate micronutrient status among term, low-birthweight, breast-fed infants in Honduras. *Journal of Nutrition*, 2004, 134:1091-1098.

77. Eneroth H et al. Duration of exclusive breast-feeding and infant iron and zinc status in rural Bangladesh. *Journal of Nutrition*, 2009, 139:1562-1567.

78. Dewey KG et al. Effects of exclusive breastfeeding for four versus six months on maternal nutritional status and infant motor development: results of two randomized trials in Honduras. *Journal of Nutrition*, 2001, 131:262-267.

79. Collins CT et al. Effect of bottles, cups, and dummies on breast feeding in preterm infants: a randomised controlled trial. *British Medical Journal*, 2004, 329:193-198.

80. Mosley C, Whittle C, Hicks C. A pilot study to assess the viability of a randomised controlled trial of methods of supplementary feeding of breast-fed pre-term babies. *Midwifery*, 2001, 17:150-157.

81. Gilks J, Watkinson M. Improving breast feeding in preterm babies: cup feeding versus bottle feeding. *Journal of Neonatal Nursing*, 2004, 10:118-120.

82. Rocha NM, Martinez FE, Jorge SM. Cup or bottle for preterm infants: effects on oxygen saturation, weight gain, and breastfeeding. *Journal of Human Lactation*, 2002, 18:132-138.

83. Marinelli KA, Burke GS, Dodd VL. A comparison of the safety of cupfeedings and bottlefeedings in premature infants whose mothers intend to breastfeed. *Journal of Perinatology*, 2001, 21:350-355.

84. Malhotra et al, A controlled trial of alternative methods of feeding in neonates. *Early Human Development*, 1999, 54:29–38.

85. Akintorin SM et al. A prospective randomized trial of feeding methods in very low birth weight infants. *Pediatrics*, 1997, 100:E4.

86. Dsilna A et al. Continuous feeding promotes gastrointestinal tolerance and growth in very low birth weight infants. *Journal of Pediatrics*, 2005, 147:43-49.

87. Toce SS, Keenan WJ, Homan SM. Enteral feeding in very-low-birth-weight infants. A comparison of two nasogastric methods. *American Journal of Diseases of Children*, 1987, 141:439-444.

88. Silvestre MA et al. A prospective randomized trial comparing continuous versus intermittent feeding methods in very low birth weight neonates. *Journal of Pediatrics*, 1996, 128:748-752.

89. Dollberg S et al. Feeding tolerance in preterm infants: randomized trial of bolus and continuous feeding. *Journal of the American College of Nutrition*, 2000, 19:797-800.

90. Stocks J. Effect of nasogastric tubes on nasal resistance during infancy. *Archives of Disease in Childhood*, 1980, 55:17-21.

91. McCormick FM, Tosh K, McGuire W. Ad libitum or demand/semi-demand feeding versus scheduled interval feeding for preterm infants. *Cochrane Database Systematic Reviews*, 2010, CD005255.

92. Kirk AT, Alder SC, King JD. Cue-based oral feeding clinical pathway results in earlier attainment of full oral feeding in premature infants. Journal of Perinatology, 2007,27:572-578.

93. Kansas KL et al. Self-regulation of feeding in the premature infant; a randomised trial of ad lib vs. scheduled feedings. *Pediatric Research*, 2004, 55: 2493.94.

94. Puckett B et al. Cue-based feeding for preterm infants: a prospective trial. *American Journal of Perinatology*, 2008, 25:623-628.

95. McCain GC et al. A feeding protocol for healthy preterm infants that shortens time to oral feeding. *Journal of Pediatrics*, 2001, 139:374-379.

96. Collinge JM et al. Demand vs. scheduled feedings for premature infants. *Journal of Obstetric, Gynecologic, and Neonatal Nursing*, 1982, 11:362–367.

97. Pridham K et al. The effects of prescribed versus ad libitum feedings and formula caloric density on premature infant dietary intake and weight gain. *Nursing Research*, 1999, 48:86–93.

98. Pridham KF et al. Comparison of caloric intake and weight outcomes of an ad lib feeding regimen for preterm infants in two nurseries. *Journal of Advanced Nursing*, 2001, 35:751-759.

99. Saunders RB, Friedman CB, Stramoski PR. Feeding preterm infants. Schedule or demand? *Journal of Obstetric, Gynecologic, and Neonatal Nursing*, 1991, 20:212–218.

100. Waber B, Hubler EG, Padden ML. A comparison of outcomes in demand versus schedule formula-fed premature infants. *Nutrition in Clinical Practice*, 1998, 13:132–135.

101. Rayyis SF et al. Randomized trial of "slow" versus "fast" feed advancements on the incidence of necrotizing enterocolitis in very low birth weight infants. *Journal of Pediatrics*, 1999, 134:293-297.

102. Salhotra A, Ramji S. Slow versus fast enteral feed advancement in very low birth weight infants: a randomized control trial. *Indian Pediatrics*, 2004, 41:435-441.

103. Krishnamurthy S et al. Slow versus rapid enteral feeding advancement in preterm newborn infants 1000-1499 g: a randomized controlled trial. *Acta Paediatrica*, 2010, 99:42-46.

104. Caple J et al. Randomized, controlled trial of slow versus rapid feeding volume advancement in preterm infants. *Pediatrics*, 2004, 114:1597-1600.